BIPOLAR
BREAKTHROUGH

BIPOLAR
BREAKTHROUGH

The Essential Guide to

Going Beyond Moodswings to

Harness Your Highs, Escape the Cycles

of Recurrent Depression,

and **Thrive with Bipolar II**

RONALD R. FIEVE, MD
best-selling author of *Moodswing*

RODALE

Rodale books may be purchased for business or promotional use or for special sales. For information, please write to:
Special Markets Department, Rodale, Inc., 733 Third Avenue, New York, NY 10017

Printed in the United States of America
Rodale Inc. makes every effort to use acid-free ♾, recycled paper ♻.

Excerpts from the *Diagnostic and Statistical Manual of Mental Disorders* on pages 44–45, 48–50, 51, 55, 58, 105, and 216–217, copyright 2000, reprinted with permission by the American Psychiatric Association.

Book design by Christina Gaugler

This revised edition was formerly published by Rodale Inc. with the title *Bipolar II*.

Library of Congress Cataloging-in-Publication Data

Fieve, Ronald R.
    Bipolar breakthrough : the essential guide to going beyond moodswings to harness your highs, escape the cycles of recurrent depression, and thrive with bipolar II / Ronald R. Fieve.
        p.   cm.
    Rev. ed. of: Bipolar II. c2006.
    Includes bibliographical references and index.
    ISBN-13 978–1–60529–645–6 paperback
    ISBN-10 1–60529–645–7 paperback
    1. Manic-depressive illness—Popular works.   2. Manic-depressive illness—Treatment—Popular works.   I. Fieve, Ronald R. Bipolar II.   II. Title.
RC516.F44   2009
616.89'5—dc22   2009020722

Distributed to the trade by Macmillan
2   4   6   8   10   9   7   5   3   1   paperback

We inspire and enable people to improve their lives and the world around them

For more of our products visit **rodalestore.com** or call 800-848-4735

To the countless volunteer patients who made the
clinical research and development of new
anti-depressive and bipolar medications possible.

To my professional staff at my private consulting office
and Fieve Clinical Services
in New York City who continue to conduct
these new investigational drug trials.

CONTENTS

FOREWORD

The clinical research field of bipolar disorders, my lifetime career, has expanded tremendously over the last 100 years since German psychiatrist Emil Kraepelin, using Falret's 1854 term "circular insanity," first employed the concept "manic-depressive insanity." Prior to this milestone, humankind suffered from nearly 2,000 years of poorly understood, inadequately labeled, and incorrectly treated psychotic behaviors.

In the early 1900s in Munich, Kraepelin—who ran the largest manic-depressive clinic in Europe of more than 1,000 patients—believed that manic depressives suffered from a biologically inherited, medically treatable defect. At the same time in Vienna, Freud was developing psychoanalysis for the treatment of neurosis, which he believed could be used to treat many cases of manic depression and schizophrenia, as well.

Kraepelin's concept of manic-depressive insanity was used by most psychiatrists during the first half of the 20th century, followed by the American Psychiatric Association's seminal first edition of the *The Diagnostic and Statistical Manual of Mental Disorders (DSM-I)* in 1952 with the new diagnostic labeling of the illness as "manic-depressive psychosis." This was later modified in the *DSM-II* edition in 1968 to the term "manic-depressive disorder," and replaced with bipolar disorder for the first time in the *DSM-III* edition, published in 1980— finally to be revised to Bipolar I and Bipolar II subtypes in the latest 1994 *DSM-IV* edition. Bipolar II indicates a milder form of the Bipolar I condition, the latter requiring at least one lifetime episode of severe mania, usually resulting in hospitalization. The breakdown of bipolar disorder into these two subtypes was based on clinical, biological, and genetic research differences among these two groups.

Subsequent research studies have found evidence for an even further breakdown of bipolar disorder into bipolar spectrum disorders, whereby subtype diagnoses of Bipolar III, Bipolar IV, and Bipolar B/Beneficial (the subject of this book) and others have been proposed for inclusion in the *DSM-V* edition, due for publication in 2012.

Subtyping a clinical psychiatric disorder enables consensus in various laboratories and psychiatric clinics around the world, where researchers can standardize their methods of investigation in order to develop specific pharmacologic/therapeutic treatments for each subtype.

With respect to the history of bipolar treatment, early Greek and Roman tents were often used as hospitals for severely disturbed bipolar patients and early treatments consisted of forced rest, restraints, projectile water therapy, and other cruel methods. Bromides were used as sedatives in the 19th century and insulin shock and electroconvulsive treatments were used extensively during the first half of the 20th century. Until the late 1950s, if none of these treatments worked, frontal lobotomy was often employed as a last resort.

In 1954, at St. Anne's hospital in Paris, the first major tranquilizer, chlorpromazine, was developed for manic depression and schizophrenia by Jean Delay and Pierre Deniker; Delay also became France's only psychiatrist ever elected to the illustrious Académie française.

Many forms of the first drug chlorpromazine were still being used to treat manic depression worldwide throughout the late '50s and '60s—even after Australian psychiatrist John Cade, in 1949, along with colleagues E. Trautner and S. Gershon, had originally discovered and used lithium as the first effective medication for manic depression. These studies were followed by Schou's confirming double-blind Danish studies in 1954 and later by the first systematic American trials of lithium that my research team and I conducted at Columbia's New York State Psychiatric Institute from 1958 on, clearly demonstrating lithium's breakthrough efficacy and its true specificity for bipolar disorder.

Today, some 60 years after its discovery, lithium remains the breakthrough treatment[1] for bipolar disorder, despite the development and use of alternative mood stabilizers and atypical antipsychotics, which have been marketed and promoted heavily. Some of these drugs have recently been shown to produce serious side effects and a generally lower efficacy than the non-promoted, non-patentable lithium. I've noted this in my bipolar practice for many years.

All bipolar experts today agree that lithium provides the highest anti-suicidal protection to the bipolar patient and the concerned family, and—when the amount present in the bloodstream is monitored closely with simple blood tests—gives maximum efficacy with the lowest incidence of side effects.

Thus, lithium remains my first choice for the treatment of most bipolar patients and it is also the least costly of all of the bipolar mood stabilizers available.

Most exciting of all is my discovery that within the bipolar spectrum also exists a beneficial creative subtype—which I have named Bipolar B—that I have observed in my practice and lithium clinics and published on since 1972.

"Most manic-depressives are not creative and most creative persons are not manic-depressive; however, when the two conditions are present simultaneously in the same individual, an incredibly creative type of human species results, and I would describe him/her as bipolar beneficial."

This discovery, along with these patients' personal case histories, is the subject of this book.

Ronald R. Fieve, MD
New York City
April 17, 2009

PART ONE

BIPOLAR II
DEFINED

CHAPTER 1

THE DECADE OF BIPOLAR II

Until recently, much of the scientific information, research, and treatments concerning manic depression were focused on Bipolar I, a major affective (that is, mood) disorder in which a person alternates between the extreme states of deep depression and intense euphoria.[1] This serious illness is characterized by elated mania with sleeplessness (often for days), hallucinations, psychosis, grandiose delusions, and/or paranoid rage. Starting in adolescence or early adulthood, Bipolar I typically persists throughout a person's life. Because of the psychotic features, those with Bipolar I almost always require hospitalization for periods of time. Well aware of Bipolar I, the general population and media have received too little information on Bipolar II, a subtype of manic depression.

I first began to notice this less-extreme version of manic depression (officially called manic-depressive psychosis at the time) in 1971 while I was in charge of the acute psychiatric service at the New York State Psychiatric Institute. Many of these milder manic-depressive patients were dynamic and industrious men and women with exuberant moods and high energy. Initially, they had come to the clinic for treatment of major depression. Yet, unlike others I had treated with manic depression, these men and women had had episodes of mildly elevated moods with high energy and tremendous productivity. In fact, these people were the proverbial "movers and shakers" of New York City. They were extremely motivated, talented, and strong-minded producers, artists, writers, musicians, doctors, lawyers, investment bankers, CEOs, sales professionals—in other words, women and men who had achieved lofty goals and the highest levels of distinction in their professional lives. Now they were sitting in front of me in my office, asking me to help stop their relentless depression.

During the years that followed, I treated literally hundreds of these mildly elated individuals for recurrent or episodic depressions—sometimes mild, but usually quite serious. Unlike their manic-depressive counterparts who alternated between extreme highs and lows, these men and women seemed to get over their depression after effective doses of antidepressants for several months, often combined with psychotherapy. During their so-called well phases, I rarely saw them.

One of these mildly elated patients whom I treated in the mid-1970s was James, who at the time was in his early twenties. The youngest of four children, he was referred to me by his sister, Susan, also a patient.

"James's personality has changed dramatically, almost overnight, and we are extremely concerned," Susan said. "Depression runs strong in our family, and James has suffered with depressed mood for almost a year.

"Recently, he became a totally different person that none of us could recognize. He hardly sleeps, and he's overly confident, flirtatious, and flamboyant, which is not like my brother at all. Also, James went with a 'hunch' last month at his securities firm and made a dreadful investment, losing more than a million dollars of his clients' money."

When James arrived at my office, he was immaculately dressed. After exchanging greetings, I asked James about his past, including his childhood and adolescent years.

"There's nothing impressive about my childhood," he said nonchalantly. "I was overweight, shy, and had few friends. In high school, I was more outgoing and was elected student body president at a private school in New England. I graduated when I was 16, and then I went to Yale on an academic scholarship to study business.

"About a year ago, I went through a horrible low period in my life," James told me. "When I sought medical care, our family doctor said it was depression and prescribed medication. I tried the drug but could not stand the way I felt. Finally, after a few weeks, I stopped the medication."

To mask his depressed feelings, James admitted that he had started drinking alcohol heavily from "breakfast until bedtime" and was using marijuana, but usually only after work or on weekends. He then told of a mystery mood transformation that had occurred over the previous month.

"Over the past couple of weeks, the depression resolved, and my mood has switched into this amazing high. I feel like I've had several cups of strong coffee, and this buzz lasts all day until late at night. I have never felt so incredible in my entire life, or had such creative ideas and high motivation," James said.

I wanted to know more about his risky investment and how he was handling the loss of a large sum of money. James brushed it off as no big deal. In fact, he was quite arrogant, remarking that no problem—even losing a million dollars—was unsolvable to him. In fact, he hinted that some insider knowledge he had on a little-known stock would more than cover the loss. And because of his "insightful brilliance," he would triple his earnings by playing the futures market over the next few months.

As I listened to James go on about his financial "genius," I could tell that he had an inflated sense of confidence with no fear of repercussions. He talked incessantly about extravagant spending on a red Jaguar, a mountain chalet in upstate New York, and wild sexual escapades that he agreed were out of character but highly enjoyable.

I recognized that James was living with a softer type of manic depression, one that we now call Bipolar II disorder. As I had observed in patients for almost a decade, this milder cyclical illness produces the enthusiasm, fervor, and incredible capacity for hard work that can be seen in many of the superachievers in our society. During the hypomanic (mildly manic) times, I saw that many of the often-brilliant high achievers were able to push themselves. It was during these times when they made the most of their ingenious ideas and productivity. But I had also witnessed a downside to this disorder, as it is accompanied by periods of bad judgment as well as episodes of deep depression, as James had experienced, that leave these men and women feeling helpless, hopeless, and worthless. When the major depression hit—and it always did—these patients usually came to see me for medication. Or if they extended too high, like James did with his investments and excessive spending, a family member or colleague would persuade them to seek medical treatment.

After talking with James for more than an hour and doing a full medical evaluation, I explained the diagnosis of this soft bipolar subtype—not yet naming it Bipolar II—and his specific treatment plan, which included stopping drinking and starting Alcoholics Anonymous (AA). All forms of bipolar disorder go hand in hand with alcoholism, and the conditions are probably related genetically. I talked with James about the ill effects of using cocaine, heroin, alcohol, marijuana, amphetamines, potentially addictive tranquilizers, and sleeping pills in an attempt to self-medicate a mood disorder.

I recommended psychotherapy to James so he could openly talk about problems that were fueling this need to drink alcohol and smoke marijuana, as well as begin to face the emotional and financial damage he had done to his personal relationships while in his hypomanic state. I then started James on a very low dose of lithium carbonate, a mood-stabilizing compound that had been approved by the FDA in 1970 for the treatment of mania in bipolar disorder. Lithium, as I'll explain further in chapter 8, is highly effective in leveling the moodswings of bipolar disorder, as well as helping to prevent future episodes.

Within a few weeks, James's mood was completely stable. He had to spend a lot of time mending fences at work and in his social life, but he was able to save his job and his reputation. Today, James is in his fifties and is still my patient. He is married with three daughters, owns a conglomerate of retail chain stores across the United States, and continues to come to my office monthly (for 30 years) to have his lithium level monitored. James also spends time periodically with a psychologist at my office, discussing any problems that may arise so he can handle them methodically and responsibly in case his moodswings threaten to dominate his thoughts and behaviors.

Within 5 years of my diagnosing James with the softer bipolar subtype, the third edition of the *Diagnostic and Statistical Manual of Mental Disorders (DSM-III)* was published in 1980 and released to the medical community. This manual, published by the American Psychiatric Association, provides physicians with diagnostic categories and criteria for making accurate diagnoses. In the third edition, the former diagnostic term "manic-depressive psychosis" was changed to "bipolar affective disorder." Over the next decade, I continued to observe periods of hypomania in bipolar patients and published my research in numerous journals. Yet it wasn't until the early 1990s that other psychiatrists and psychopharmacologists also began to catch on and differentiate between Bipolar I and Bipolar II disorder. (A psychopharmacologist is a psychiatrist who is an expert in using medications to treat psychiatric chemical imbalances.) In 1994, the American Psychiatric Association officially recognized the differences between Bipolar I and Bipolar II in the fourth edition of the *DSM (DSM-IV)*. Since then, the national media have reported on Bipolar II, and terms such as "hypomanic" are now regularly used in the medical community.

3 Feelings of Depression

1. Helpless
2. Hopeless
3. Worthless

HOW THIS BOOK CAN HELP

Despite the increasing attention Bipolar II disorder has been given since I first began diagnosing it, most psychiatrists and primary care physicians today vastly underuse the diagnosis of this softer bipolar disorder. In fact, it is not uncommon for a patient to see four or five doctors before coming to my office and finally obtaining the proper diagnosis of Bipolar II and effective treatment—or *no treatment at all.* When I speak before manic-depressive support groups, at medical gatherings, or consult with patients, it surprises me that so many patients and their families are still unaware of Bipolar II disorder and assume that all manic depression falls into the category of Bipolar I with its wildly manic psychosis and devastating depressions. But I continue to educate patients, physicians, and the population about the wide variations in mood and the high prevalence of Bipolar II disorder, hoping that some day it will not be thought of simply as a serious form of bipolar illness, but rather accepted as a potentially beneficial condition with enormous advantages.

As you read through this book, you will see that it quickly moves beyond a discussion of Bipolar I and Bipolar II disorders and on to page after page of groundbreaking medical studies and real patient stories, describing how Bipolar II manifests itself with its exuberant hypomania and how this disorder is diagnosed and treated.

Here's how I'll accomplish this.

In part one, Bipolar II Defined, I will give you the full

description of Bipolar II, from the signs and symptoms to sleep problems to more serious outcomes such as hypersexuality and financial ruin. Starting in this chapter, The Decade of Bipolar II, I'll introduce you to Bipolar I with its wild mania and psychotic hallucinations and explain how it differs from Bipolar II, with its episodes of major depression and mild mania or hypomania. The real patient stories are intriguing and will help you fully grasp the wide range of moods and symptoms that frequently occur with this common mood disorder.

Chapter 2, The Bipolar Spectrum at a Glance, is perhaps the most important chapter in the book as I focus on the wide range of moodswings that can occur in the bipolar spectrum and specific criteria psychiatrists use for making a diagnosis.

You'll learn about the link between your family tree and Bipolar II in chapter 3, Moodswing and Family Genetics. I will describe celebrities and ordinary patients who have realized the bipolar linkage in their family trees, as well as the latest journal studies linking Bipolar II to other behaviors such as attention-deficit/hyperactivity disorder (ADHD), alcoholism, depression, gambling, and even high achievement.

Sleep and biological rhythms are the focus of discussion in chapter 4. Through years of clinical trials with bipolar patients, I have found that the lack of need for sleep—referred to as the hypomanic alert—oftentimes initiates a hypomanic phase and is absolutely critical in making an accurate diagnosis of most Bipolar IIs. I will discuss the lack of sleep and Bipolar II more extensively in chapter 4 and give you and your family some self-help strategies.

I believe that chapter 5, Sex, Drugs, and Other (Mis)behaviors, will open your eyes to some risky patterns associated with Bipolar II disorder. While not everyone who has Bipolar II is hypersexual, abuses drugs or alcohol, and has financial indiscretions, it is important to be aware of these frequently co-occurring behaviors. You and your family can take steps early on to avoid high-risk situations and an impending crisis.

While bipolar disorder traditionally has had a negative connotation, I will educate you about some extremely positive aspects of this disorder in chapter 6, The Hypomanic Advantage of Bipolar II Beneficial. I coined the term "hypomanic edge" and talked about it on the *Today* show with Barbara Walters in the mid-1970s after realizing that about 50 percent of my Bipolar II patients were some of the most successful high achievers in New York City. I'll discuss the hypomanic advantages I have identified and elaborate on how these attributes can be used to improve the patient's life, as well as impact society as a whole.

In part two, Diagnosis and Treatment of Bipolar II, I will explain how this disorder is diagnosed and treated and help you gain insight into specific situations such as pregnancy, when doctors, patients, and families must work closely together for the best outcome.

In chapter 7, The Bipolar II Consultation, I'll elaborate on the various questions I usually ask patients when they come for the initial consultation and explain the medical protocol used for making the diagnosis, including blood chemistries, electrocardiogram (ECG), chest x-ray, and urinalysis, among other tests.

Treatment varies with Bipolar II disorder and in chapter 8, Modulating Moods, I will give you the history of my pioneering studies with lithium in the United States. I'll also discuss other mood stabilizers and medications commonly used today and give you further insight into effects and side effects.

There are certain stages in the life cycle, such as pregnancy, childhood, or the elderly years, when patients and doctors must work closely to find safe and effective treatment for moodswings. I will explain these delicate life stages in chapter 9, Special Situations That Complicate a Bipolar Diagnosis, and also give new insight into diagnosing and treating children and adolescents with ADHD and/or Bipolar II disorder.

Chapter 10, Stay-Well Strategies, simplifies all you've learned throughout this book. In this chapter I will provide you and your family with easy suggestions on how to monitor mood each day so you can notify the doctor before there is a more serious problem. I will suggest ways to keep your lifestyle habits balanced to prevent wide variations in mood, and I will encourage you and your family to stay positive and resilient to have the best outcome. I realize that being diagnosed with a mood disorder is a tremendous challenge to patients and their families, and I wrote this last chapter to give you ultimate hope and support.

So that you derive the greatest benefit from this book, I recommend starting with this first chapter and carefully reading each subsequent chapter to the end of the book. But if you are seeking information on a specific concern such as sleep problems, pregnancy, or medications, go ahead and turn to the chapters that discuss these topics. You can then come back to chapter 1 and begin reading the book from start to completion. Lastly, if you or a family member has recently been diagnosed with Bipolar II, I urge you to turn to chapter 6, The Hypomanic Advantage of Bipolar II Beneficial, and learn about the gifted attributes or benefits that are often associated with Bipolar II. Over the past 3 decades, I've repeatedly found that when patients are aware of these extraordinary gifts, their inner confidence is boosted and they are more likely to be compliant to healthy lifestyle habits such as getting quality sleep each night and avoiding alcohol. Because the patients feel better, they also check in with me regularly to make sure their mood is stabilized and report problems early on, when treatment is most effective.

By starting now to learn more about Bipolar II disorder, you can protect your emotional health and the health of your loved ones. To that end, this first chapter gives you the necessary groundwork to understand this intriguing but often complicated mood disorder, and it will set the stage for the rest of this book.

WHAT IS BIPOLAR DISORDER?

Bipolar disorder is a complex genetic disorder characterized by dramatic or unusual moodswings between major depression and extreme elation, accompanied by disturbances in thinking, distortions of perception, and impairment in social functioning. The moodswings of bipolar disorder can range from very mild to extreme and can come on gradually or suddenly within minutes to hours. There are two subtypes of bipolar disorder:

1. Those patients with Bipolar I disorder who have a history of at least one manic episode, with or without past major depressive episodes.
2. Those patients with Bipolar II disorder who have a history of at least one episode of major depression and at least one hypomanic episode.

As a point of reference, throughout this book I will sometimes refer to "bipolar disorder," meaning both Bipolar I and Bipolar II and the spectrum of symptoms I'll discuss in chapter 2. But when I speak of the specific subtypes, I will qualify each as either Bipolar I or Bipolar II.

The age of onset of bipolar disorder is usually between ages 17 and 29 years.[2] Newly diagnosed mania rarely occurs in children or in adults over the age of 65.[3] Although the cause is not fully understood, it is now thought that there is a strong genetic component to bipolar disorder.

Marked by relapses and remissions, bipolar disorder has a high rate of recurrence if untreated. At the turn of the century, the famous German psychiatrist Emil Kraepelin, often called the Father of Psychiatry, found in his Munich clinic that the average period of feeling "well" after a mood episode was:

- 4.3 years after the first episode
- 2.8 years after the second episode
- 1.8 years after the third episode
- 1.7 years after the fourth episode
- 1.5 years after the fifth episode

Over the years, I have repeatedly seen that after the first Bipolar II episode, there is usually a guaranteed downward spiral in the patient's personal life as hypomanic or depressive symptoms skyrocket. One mood episode is usually accepted, and employers and family members trust that the patient will seek professional medical attention for the problem. But, again, as I've experienced, most patients initially ignore treatment and experience a second episode of hypomania or fall into a major depression, rendering them unable to work or function, and then they usually lose their jobs. The third episode of hypomania or depression, which is often more intense and occurs sooner than the second one did, may result in a spouse leaving or family members turning away from the person altogether. As life progresses and episodes recur without stabilization, the prognosis for unmanaged moodswings is not nearly so good as with the first episode. That is why education, early diagnosis, and effective treatment of the Bipolar II patient with medications that stabilize moods prevent the worsening of the illness that would otherwise occur.

You're probably thinking, "Hey, there's no way that I could have Bipolar II disorder. I just have more energy and need less sleep than most people my age." Few individuals think they have Bipolar II disorder, especially with all the negative press this mood disorder has received over the past few years.

But while bipolar disorder was once thought to affect about 1 percent of the population, we now believe that the lifetime prevalence may be much higher than previously thought, although without laboratory tests to substantiate the diagnosis, it can be misdiagnosed, depending on the clinician. The expert consensus is that the chance of developing a manic, hypomanic, or depressive episode in a lifetime could be as high as 6.5 percent of the population,[4] or about 1 person in 15. But as common as it might be, it is thought that about 80 percent of those people with bipolar tendencies have not been evaluated by a psychiatrist nor have they been diagnosed, and nearly one-third of patients are misdiagnosed with unipolar depression or major depression without the mania or hypomania.

Historical Perspective of the Diagnostic Term "Bipolar Disorder"

1958: *DSM-I* included manic depression as a legitimate diagnosis.

1968: *DSM-II* changed the term from manic depression to manic-depressive psychosis, wherein people swing back and forth between depression and mania.

1980: *DSM-III* changed the diagnostic term manic-depressive psychosis to bipolar affective disorder.

1994: For the first time, *DSM-IV* subdivided manic depression into Bipolar I and Bipolar II, along with detailing the difference in symptom patterns.

BIPOLAR I AND MANIA

Before you can fully comprehend Bipolar II, it is important that you understand Bipolar I, which is characterized by episodes of mania, usually following an episode of mild to major depression—but not always. With the mania, the person is abnormally elated, energetic, and extremely talkative for at least a week or longer. The episodic mania can also be violent, agitated, and paranoid so that the patient injures himself or loved ones. Some patients go so high during a manic state that they believe God is sending them secret messages through the television set about a mission they are to fulfill on Earth. One Bipolar I patient of mine, while in a manic state, actually left his home in Greenwich, Connecticut, one night during the late news, drove to New York City in his bathrobe and slippers, and was arrested by police after trying to break into a local television studio through a back window. His intent? He said the young woman reporter was making gestures to him during the newscast to secretly meet her at the station. He was a man on a mission but, sadly, the mission was all in his markedly manic mind.

Patients with Bipolar I mania, such as my Connecticut patient, usually require hospitalization to keep them from engaging in risky behaviors. Those who are severely depressed also might need hospitalization to keep them from acting on suicidal thoughts. About 90 percent of individuals with Bipolar I disorder have at least one psychiatric hospitalization, and two-thirds have two or more hospitalizations in their lifetimes.[5]

Of course, full-blown mania is undeniably recognizable to most people, yet the afflicted person is usually unaware that anything is wrong with them at all. Take Carole as an example. I had treated this 23-year-old legal assistant previously for an eating disorder and two depressive episodes. A bright and attractive young woman, Carole had been soft-spoken and reserved when she had come to my office, and, at the time, she had no signs of mania.

It wasn't until her older sister, Anna, with whom she shared an apartment in New York City, called me on my cell phone at about 6:00 a.m. that I was alerted to Carole's severe mood-swing. "We have a problem, and I need your help," Anna said. "Carole is acting extremely paranoid. She claims she's searching for someone who is trying to break into our house."

I thought that Carole might be having a manic episode, which is usually characterized by anger and paranoia or even euphoria. Given the young woman's history of eating disorders and depressive episodes, the mania would indicate that she had Bipolar I, which almost always requires medication and even hospitalization to stabilize the mood.

Anna continued, "For the past few days, she has spent hours carving these deep holes in our oak cabinets and then she saves the wood shavings in a locked box under her bed. I hear her roaming the house at all hours during the night, and she has not gone to work this week. Last night Carole seemed very agitated, which is unlike her. When I walked into the living room to turn off the light, she was hiding behind the drapes and motioned for me to hide, too. She told me she heard something in the walls.

I did not say anything because it was too odd and, quite honestly, her behavior frightened me. So I sat on the couch and waited until she went into the kitchen, where, again, she got her little knife and began to carve tiny holes in the kitchen cabinets. It's completely bizarre, watching Carole dig holes in our cabinets as if she really might find something or someone.

"I then went to the den to watch television. I knew I needed to call for help but at the time could not think of whom to call. I had just dozed off during the late-night news when Carole came in the den, stood behind my recliner, and began screaming that I had to stop talking to our parents using the television remote control. It was like a nightmare, and our parents are deceased! When I turned around, Carole's eyes were very glassy, almost trancelike, and she was staring at the TV remote like it held some kind of power. I had never seen Carole act this way before. That's when I remembered that she had seen you last year for depression."

I urged Anna to bring Carole to my office immediately. Most Bipolar I patients refuse to see a doctor during a manic episode, but Anna thought Carole would be agreeable as she had seen me previously.

As I observed Carole later that morning, I could see that she was in a highly physically agitated and frenzied state with her eyes darting around the room. She was extremely talkative (called pressured speech), and many of her words were garbled and even rhymed, making no sense to me. She was greatly distracted when I asked her questions. But when her eyes fixated on my computer mouse, and I could not break her stare, I knew she was not in a normal mood state.

I explained to Carole that I thought she was experiencing a manic episode associated with Bipolar I disorder, where the moodswings range from depression to mania. With Anna's support, we convinced Carole to start antipsychotic medication immediately to avoid having to be admitted to the hospital. If she did have to go to the hospital, she would be admitted to the psychiatric unit for observation and treatment.

Surprisingly, Carole was compliant and agreed to take the antipsychotic medication. Anna vowed to watch Carole to make sure the medication was taken as scheduled. She said she would call my office daily to give me a progress report on her sister.

It took about a week for the medication to bring Carole's mood state back to normal. At the follow-up visit, Carole was back to her usual reserved self and had little recollection of the manic episode, which is not uncommon for those with Bipolar I. She set up a series of appointments to check in with me each week and then every 2 weeks for a while to make sure the medication dosage was correct and without serious side effects. Carole took a leave of absence from her job and was able to go back to work full-time—and on medication—in 2 months. Today she remains on the medication and is diligent about keeping her appointments with me.

In psychotic mania, the most severe form of mania, the Bipolar I person may hallucinate or have grandiose religious or paranoid delusions like Carole's. When this happens, the fully manic person almost always refuses medical treatment because they do not perceive that they are ill. I cannot tell you how many manic Bipolar I patients have told the admitting doctor at the emergency room that the quite normal persons who brought them to the hospital were "out of their minds"—not them. If severe mania goes untreated, however, there is the risk of full psychosis and collapse brought on by physical and mental exhaustion. At that time, hospitalization is necessary and must be made at the request of the family and, oftentimes, the local police. So many times, the hospitalization of a psychotic manic person has to be forced legally, whereby two psychiatrists must agree that the patient presents a threat to himself or to others in the community.

BIPOLAR II'S HYPOMANIA AND DEPRESSION

While mania is the feature characteristic of Bipolar I, Bipolar II has milder periods of elation, or hypomania, along with episodes of mild or major depression. The difference between mania and hypomania is one of degree, or according to the *DSM-IV*, "the degree of severity." Both mania and hypomania exhibit grandiose mood and reduced need for sleep, but these characteristics are milder in hypomania. Also, hypomania is a far more productive, active period that is usually associated with highly successful individuals—those who are highly ambitious overachievers and entrepreneurs. That said, it is important to note that not everyone who is enthusiastic and highly driven and who moves quickly is hypomanic. There are many high-spirited superachievers who are exceedingly productive, successful, and need little sleep but who also have normal moods that do not affect their daily activities, decision making, or relationships.

If you've had times when you were incredibly energetic, charming, garrulous, and persuasive, perhaps you have a tendency toward hypomania. The hypomanic person is the fast-talking "million-dollar" salesman who moves to the top of his field seemingly overnight; the exuberant politician who has yet to taste defeat; the Stepford Wife "super mom" who juggles a high-powered corporate position with raising brilliant children and chairing community fund-raisers while getting by on 3 hours of sleep each night. Charismatic, vivacious, and dynamic, the hypomanic man or woman outranks others in the same field—until he or she tastes the other side of hypomania and becomes irritable, angry, arrogant, and even paranoid or falls low into a major depressive episode with fatigue, feelings of worthlessness or guilt, impaired concentration, and even recurring thoughts of suicide.

If you met Sophia, you'd probably be surprised to find out she had Bipolar II disorder with its episodes of hypomania and major depression. This young woman is brilliant, gorgeous, and highly successful as an attorney. She'd graduated from a prestigious Ivy League law school, been an editor on the Law Review, and clerked for a federal judge in New York. Sophia took pride in her high achievements and unusual productivity. Several members of her family were also high achievers and had the same energy. She was widely recognized as a rising star, both inordinately driven and disciplined.

Right after she graduated from law school, Sophia took a brief vacation with friends in the Caribbean. Upon returning, this normally sensible and well-spoken young woman said that she awoke one day in her Manhattan loft feeling hyperalert, sexier, and smarter than before. At work, she felt as if she could concentrate much better. Where before she'd slept 8 hours a night, she suddenly found her thoughts racing, and she slept only 3 hours, with no daytime fatigue. She felt she had become a "powerhouse." After working 15-hour days for weeks on end and studying for the New York bar exam, Sophia was going out every night and enjoying the mild elation of the SoHo club scene. Friends mentioned that she was more talkative, animated, and outgoing, and she was enjoying her increased attraction to the opposite sex, bringing different men back to her apartment each night. She also began spending money recklessly, buying a diamond tennis bracelet and a high-definition television, as well as dozens of articles of clothing, which were provocative.

After about 2 months on this manic ride, Sophia crashed. She felt apathetic and fatigued, and had no appetite or grandiose ideas. She also failed to see any joy in the pricey stuff she had charged to her credit card. Her body felt lifeless, heavy, and fatigued, and she just wanted to sleep. It wasn't until she failed to show up for work—or even call in—3 days in a row that her roommate insisted she make an appointment at my office. Her roommate was aware of the dramatic changes in Sophia's moods and behavior, and knew that she needed help.

In my office, Sophia told me her family history, which revealed that her family was a typical one for people with bipolar disorder.

"My mother had severe depression for years and was diagnosed late in life as having a recurrent major depressive disorder,"

Sophia said. "My uncle (my mom's brother) committed suicide at age 24."

Sophia went on to tell about her younger sister, who appeared to have dysthymia (from the Greek "bad" and "mood"), a chronically depressed mood that occurs for most of the day, more days than not, for at least 2 years. A person with dysthymia seems to function normally but actually feels unhappy most of the time, or always below par. Sophia's older brother was an alcoholic and had been in rehab twice in the past year. Sophia's maternal grandmother had had a history of "going to bed for weeks at a time," she recalled. As a child, Sophia had been told that her grandmother was just "sad and tired."

After listening to Sophia's lengthy family history, it seemed to me that she had a strong bipolar heritage. Many bipolar families have members who are extremely successful like Sophia, along with those relatives who are alcohol or drug abusers, depressed, suicidal, gamblers, etc. After explaining the bipolar family "portrait" to Sophia, we talked at length about her hypomanic mood and the resulting behaviors—the impulsive and pricey shopping spree, the decreased need for sleep, and the increased sex drive. We also discussed her bout with major depression, and the increased need for sleep, as well as feelings of hopelessness, sadness, and emptiness.

I diagnosed Sophia with Bipolar II, and as with many of my patients, I found that a small dose of a commonly used anticonvulsant, along with an antidepressant, worked to stabilize the young woman's moods. As often happens when a patient gets a diagnosis of bipolar disorder, Sophia initially exhibited a great deal of anger and denial. She said the diagnosis was "bogus," and she was going to seek another professional opinion immediately. She then questioned how she could have been so successful in law school if she had a psychiatric illness. As we talked, she began to express fears, such as how this illness would affect her career as a lawyer. And what about marriage and children—could she still have healthy children with this genetic linkage? I listened to Sophia's utmost concerns and then assured her that in part because of the Bipolar II hypomania, she had risen to the top in law school and would continue to be a highly effective and persuasive attorney and successful young woman. The elated and energetic hypomanic mood would most likely help her win clients as well as the jury verdict in the courtroom. I also gave her a referral to a genetic counselor at Columbia University, so she could talk with this professional about the genetics of bipolar illness.

Sophia continued to come to my office weekly and then monthly for the remainder of the year, and her moods remained stable on medication. She worked closely with a psychologist in my office as she learned more about Bipolar II disorder, and eventually she began to accept the diagnosis and talk openly about it with family and friends. She eventually got engaged to another attorney, went to genetic counseling with her fiancé, and then moved to upstate New York after getting married. She made plans to find a new psychiatrist and continue her treatments, which she would need to avoid going too high and possibly spiraling into a Bipolar II major depressive episode again.

The Upside of Hypomania

Until the 1990s, mania had been viewed as an emotional illness only in its most conspicuous form—the often dangerous and self-destructive highs of an extreme manic episode with the psychosis that is characteristic of Bipolar I. The milder highs associated with Bipolar II had gone largely unnoticed, mainly because the person experiencing them finds these between-depression phases not only a welcome relief but also a time of tremendous energy and mild elation. I strongly believe that the hypomanic phase may at times be of great benefit to the patient and often to society as well. During these mild highs, the patient refers to the "up" mood as feeling normal, so why try to fix it?

An example of this is Whitney. After I diagnosed this

28-year-old woman with Bipolar II disorder, she immediately responded, "No medication allowed." This vivacious, ebullient pharmaceutical sales rep did not find the hypomanic mood problematic in any way and certainly did not want it "squelched with medication."

"I crave my upbeat mood and unending energy level," Whitney said to me. "That's how I've made it to the top of my field so fast."

While Whitney admitted that she often went on shopping sprees that were a bit outrageous and way out of line with her budget, they were exciting and made her feel affluent. This young woman especially enjoyed her hypersexuality, although she did worry that she might have some problems if her disorder led to a lack of judgment and she became too promiscuous. For now, she was in a monogamous relationship, so her heightened sexual behavior was not a personal concern.

I spoke frankly with Whitney about Bipolar II disorder and how sometimes the hypomanic "good feeling" can cause people to make impulsive decisions that they might later regret. She promised to stay in touch with me and let me know if her behavior changed in such a way as to indicate that her mood was going too high. She also agreed to educate her boyfriend on Bipolar II disorder and ask him to help monitor her moods. So many times, it is another family member or close friend who is first aware of the Bipolar II patient going too high. I always tell patients that medications can usually stabilize the hypomanic mood without interfering with their lifestyle and daily activities, but they need to come in when they first notice a problem.

Perhaps the most reliable predictor of hypomania is the amount of sleep a person requires. Whitney, for example, got between 3 and 4 hours each night and never stopped to take a catnap or break. I'd wager that someone who gets 3, maybe 4, hours of sleep a night is hypomanic. This person usually has no complaints about insomnia and does not need to catch up on lost sleep. Usually, the hypomanic individual shows antipathy toward sleep, considering it to be a complete waste of time! And most highly ambitious hypomanic patients, like my patient Keith, age 49, make this lack of sleep work for them.

Five nights each week, Keith works the night shift at a local hospital emergency room in patient admissions. During the day-time hours, he works full-time at a public relations agency and is a senior account representative for several national car dealer-ships. Keith goes nonstop from his day job to his nighttime work and then catches a few hours of sleep in between. During two major depressive episodes over the past 12 years, he did stop his night job because his need for sleep greatly increased. But when his Bipolar II hypomanic state returned, Keith went back to both jobs and was once again highly visible around New York City in his dual careers and social life.

Most hypomanic men and women are very self-motivated and have what I call the entrepreneurial personality. In fact, a high percentage of the entrepreneurs I've studied have Bipolar II disorder, which may explain their attraction to entrepreneurship in the first place. They have this strong inner drive or stimulus that motivates them to work harder, be more productive, achieve more, and also snap back quickly if life's interruptions or busi-ness setbacks block their paths. They are restless, impatient, and oftentimes harbor racing thoughts on how they will accomplish the next venture, build their empire, or create the next family dynasty.

You might say that hypomanics crave the "fast lane" in life. They think fast, talk fast, and dominate conversations with family, friends, and colleagues, sometimes interrupting everyone because their "great idea" must be of more importance than the conversation at hand.

The Downside of Hypomania

It is easy for those with Bipolar II to romanticize the hypomanic mood until they experience compulsive gambling or financial loss, impulsivity, hypersexuality, or substance abuse—all behaviors commonly found in those with Bipolar II. Bipolar II's hypomania can generally make a person feel vivacious and exhilarated, but it can also make that same person increasingly haughty, ill-tempered, and difficult to be around; not all is rosy when you're wearing a Bipolar II "happy face." An exuberant, glowing Bipolar II will usually seek medical help only when the moodswing and resulting behavior go too far and judgment becomes skewed, resulting in irrational behavior, or when the much-dreaded crash of major depression occurs. I've seen numerous hypomanics who overestimate their abilities, and while their minds are sharp, their judgment is sometimes poor, resulting in impulsive decision-making, job loss, reduced income, broken relationships, and even suicide.

Sometimes the Bipolar II hypomania goes too high, which becomes evident in increased physical activity and more rapid and irritable speech. The elated disposition becomes hostile and angry, resulting in explosive words and actions. A case in point is Alicia, who blames hypomania (not herself) for causing her three divorces. This 39-year-old high school English teacher and symphony harpist is perhaps one of the most brilliant and eloquent women I have ever treated.

Common Signs of Hypomania

- Exuberant and elated mood
- Increased confidence
- Extremely focused on projects at work or at home
- Increased creativity and productivity
- Decreased need for sleep
- Increased energy and libido
- Risk-taking behaviors
- Reckless behaviors

"Most of the time, I can control my moods by taking medication and getting a lot of exercise and eating balanced meals," Alicia said. "But almost invariably after a mild depressive episode, I start to feel overly confident and very self-assured. I always think I'm 'cured' of the mood disorder and stop taking my medication. This invariably sends me into a hypomanic spiral that results in little sleep and a quick, sharp tongue that lashes out at family and friends."

I've explained to Alicia, as I have with all of my patients, that there is no need for the negative feelings associated with Bipolar II to ruin your life. If personal feelings and behaviors are out of control and interfering with your daily living, job, and relationships, then we need to rethink the medications and find the exact one that effectively stabilizes the mood without causing uncomfortable side effects. Alicia now stays on a low dose of a mood stabilizer, works with a staff psychologist on ways to change past destructive behaviors, and is learning effective communication skills that can help in establishing meaningful long-term relationships.

I often compare the milder Bipolar II disorder to a double-edged sword. The hypercompetency and adaptation in creative and productive hypomanics are of inestimable value. But when one extends too high and becomes too irritable or haughty, like Alicia, the biological disadvantage becomes apparent. If a hypomanic swings into depression, the other edge of the sword is exposed. The Jekyll and Hyde transformations of Bipolar II can be painful and totally disruptive to everyone. One cannot rely on the consistency of mood changes since the bipolar illness often takes on a life of its own. Most Bipolar II hypomanics in the public eye or in high corporate positions have guaranteed valleys of major depression and periods of inactivity. Hospitalization for "fatigue," or mysterious trips out of town with no forwarding number, may be the only clues to those around them that something is seriously wrong.

Over the past few decades, I have come to realize that no

one needs to live with volatile moodswings. Most depressive episodes associated with Bipolar II are treatable with the right combination of medication and psychotherapy. There is also treatment for hypomania if the exuberance extends too far into irritability, rage, or poor judgment.

Still, I could describe hundreds of patients I have treated who are extremely hard to persuade to come in for treatment during the exhilarating hypomania. This is true even when they are impulsively destroying their careers, marriages, finances, and reputations because of their out-of-control mood state. Why should you go to see Dr. Fieve (or any psychiatrist or psychopharmacologist) when you're highly productive, energetic, and creative? I mean, most people would love to be so industrious and intuitive! And hypomanics are usually their most successful selves—or their worst destructive enemies—during these high moods.

EARLY DIAGNOSIS IS IMPORTANT

I cannot tell you the number of messages I get from patients (and even non-patients) who ask me to please call in medication for their "self-diagnosed" depression, a dangerous practice if the psychiatrist is not carefully monitoring the patient weekly, biweekly, or monthly. A few months ago, a gentleman I'll call Daniel left a message that said, "Dr. Fieve, I am feeling horribly depressed and need something to boost my mood fast before I leave on vacation. Would you please call in some Prozac or Wellbutrin [two popular antidepressants]?" Ironically, Daniel, who had just finished reading my first book, *Moodswing*, was not even my patient!

Today's medical environment is characterized by "quick fixes," and a person like Daniel complaining of depression without mentioning periods of hypomania or other symptoms can easily be misdiagnosed and recklessly medicated. I tell my patients up front that diagnosing and treating mood disorders is not a black and white process, and there is an art to identifying the specific disorder and then finding the precise medications to stabilize each patient, while allowing them to continue to function at the highest level possible. According to a recent survey by the National Depressive and Manic Depressive Association (NDMDA), patients go an average of 8 to 10 years without receiving an accurate diagnosis and effective medical treatment.[5] Because the symptoms of depression and hypomania are sometimes similar to other psychiatric disorders, bipolar patients often get the inaccurate diagnosis of dysthymic (formerly called neurotic) depression, personality disorder, attention-deficit/hyperactivity disorder (ADHD), and generalized anxiety disorder, among others. In addition, a medical condition such as stroke or hypothyroidism may have symptoms that mimic bipolar disorder, or there can be corticosteroid-induced symptoms, when a steroid medication is given in higher doses to resolve inflammation in diseases such as asthma or rheumatoid arthritis.

There are millions of underdiagnosed Bipolar IIs who are routinely prescribed tranquilizers and sleeping pills by their primary care physicians instead of being referred to a mood disorder specialist (either a psychiatrist or psychopharmacologist) who can make an accurate diagnosis and prescribe the correct combination of medication and/or cognitive therapy. Because of poor training in medical school, most general practitioners diagnose Bipolar II disorder as "anxiety" or "depression," instead of realizing that it is a very specific mood disorder that mandates proper treatment. Patients may suffer needlessly for years with erroneous treatments that numb brilliant minds, compromise their creativity, and deprive them of intimate relationships, successful careers, and overall quality of life.

Because patients with Bipolar II seek treatment for the "low moods" and not the hypomania, it makes sense that depression is more likely to be recognized and treated. The problem with prescribing antidepressants is that in some people who are susceptible to bipolar disorder, the medication can precipitate hypomania or mania, even if the person has no prior history of this mood state. I will further explain this medication-induced personality transformation called Bipolar III in chapter 2, but for now just be aware of this fact and make sure you always know your personal medical and family history before you accept a doctor's recommendation to take an antidepressant medication.

With Bipolar II, it is common to have coexisting conditions (one or more psychiatric or medical disorders that co-occur with the illness) that can complicate the diagnosis and treatment. For example, it's not uncommon for the Bipolar II patient to also have coexisting generalized anxiety disorder, panic attacks, phobias, social anxiety, conduct disorders, eating disorders, substance abuse, sexual addiction, ADHD, and problems with impulse control, among others. I will address these conditions throughout the book.

Without proper diagnosis and treatment, a person may subsequently suffer more frequent and/or severe hypomanic and depressive episodes (called rapid-cycling) than those experienced when the signs and symptoms first appeared. The episodes following often occur sooner and more spontaneously. The succeeding episodes usually last longer and may be less responsive to treatment because of the comorbid conditions that begin to develop and the disintegration of the family support system and/or difficulties at work. Some patients even develop treatment-resistant bipolar disorder, or their treatment may become ineffective with alcohol or substance abuse. Many patients stop treatment altogether, oftentimes within weeks after taking the medication, which can result in the mood soaring too high or falling too low, accompanied by suicidal ideation. Bipolarity has the highest suicide rate of all mental illnesses—an extraordinary 10 to 20 percent of untreated bipolar patients, as estimated by the National Institute of Mental Health. However, in a number of studies, lithium treatment, when compared to all other mood-stabilizing drugs, has consistently proven to be the most anti-suicidal drug for bipolar disorders.[7]

UNDERSTANDING BRINGS HOPE

I believe that Bipolar II, with its intrinsically pleasurable hypomania and softer moodswings, is vastly becoming the new diagnosis of the decade for a large part of our culture. Most people crave the energetic, creative, and exuberant side of this milder form of bipolar disorder, especially in our frenzied society where men and women are propelled to early success by working 70- to 80-hour weeks. I bet if I evaluated the mental health of the top 10 most successful men and women in America, most—*if not all*—would have this milder form of bipolar disorder with the distinct hypomanic mood.

That said, the most important point I want to make in writing this book is what we can achieve if we properly recognize and effectively treat Bipolar II. I cannot stress enough how confident and encouraged I feel about this possibility. Not only do the patients stand to benefit from proper treatment that keeps them running at the top of their game, but society will continue to be enhanced by their incredible creativity, productivity, and achievements.

For Those with Bipolar II and Their Family Members

■ Review the facts about Bipolar I and Bipolar II as discussed in this chapter, and talk about moodswings with family members, friends, and co-workers and/or employer. Openness, education, and acceptance are crucial to avoid problems associated with Bipolar II disorder, particularly when the mood elevates too high or falls into a depression. Whereas someone with Bipolar II might not be aware of the mildly elevated mood changes, an intuitive family member or friend can recognize these subtle changes and talk to the person or his or her physician before the mood extends too far.

■ Understand the differences between Bipolar I and Bipolar II disorder and talk to your doctor if you feel you have been misdiagnosed. You may be overly medicated, wrongly medicated, or need no medication at all.

■ Seek a second opinion from a specialist (psychiatrist or psychopharmacologist) if you have doubts about your current medications.

■ Work with the specialist to find the best treatment regimen with the fewest side effects. It usually takes several tries with different medications to find the right one or best combination of medications that work best for you. If no medication is recommended, use healthy lifestyle habits, particularly getting ample sleep and regular exercise, to keep moods balanced.

■ If your mood interferes with your daily activities, career, and relationships, then it is important to talk to a medical professional who fully understands Bipolar II disorder and the way it can manifest in different people and find out if different treatment is necessary.

■ Take opportunities to use the highly creative and productive side of a Bipolar II disorder both at home and at work to increase feelings of self-worth and confidence.

THE BIPOLAR SPECTRUM AT A GLANCE

Bipolar disorder is one of the most common and clearly defined, yet one of the most baffling emotional disorders. For instance, the Bipolar I person may seem normal for months—even years—and then suddenly enter a period of elated mania in which he or she stays awake all night, is hypersexual, hears voices that are not real, and swings from invisible chandeliers (sometimes literally). After returning to a normal mood state, for no apparent reason, the person may then wake up in a deep depression and even become suicidal.

I have been intrigued by bipolar disorder since I first started my psychiatric studies at Harvard Medical School. At that time, very little was understood about this illness, which manifests itself in distinct moodswings ranging from wildly frenzied mania to extremely despondent depression, and Bipolar I patients were often "tossed into the schizophrenia wastebasket," resulting in years of inappropriate treatment and unnecessary suffering for the patient and family. Later, when I did my residency at the New York State Psychiatric Institute at Columbia Presbyterian Medical Center in New York City, psychiatrists had just started using psychoactive drugs such as the antipsychotic phenothiazine tranquilizer Thorazine (chlorpromazine) to chemically treat highly agitated patients with schizophrenia and Bipolar I. And, for the first time in a hundred years, the number of patients admitted to psychiatric hospitals began to decline.

Since my studies at Harvard and Columbia, the understanding of and treatment for bipolar disorders have dramatically changed. Not only is bipolar disorder fully documented and broken down into two subtypes (Bipolar I and Bipolar II) in the *DSM-IV,* but there are a limited number of newly developed medications available to successfully modulate the highs and lows of these illnesses, as well as prevent future episodes. When properly diagnosed and treated with medications and psychotherapy, it is possible for 70 to 80 percent of those with bipolar disorder to lead a normal and extremely productive life. Still, it is estimated that two out of three people with bipolar disorder do not get proper treatment because their moods are not recognized, or they are misdiagnosed.

In this chapter, I will introduce the link between chemical messengers in the brain called neurotransmitters and how they affect your mood, causing you to feel happy, anxious, sad, or depressed. Over the past several decades, scientists have learned a great deal about these brain chemicals and have developed highly specific medications, such as the newer antidepressants, that work to normalize them. As you move through the chapter, I will introduce the wide range of moods and feelings on the bipolar spectrum and the corresponding signs and symptoms. A full understanding of these signs and symptoms can alert you to a potential problem and allow you to speak with your doctor for a proper diagnosis and treatment, if necessary, before the mood escalates.

NEUROTRANSMITTERS, MOOD, AND DEPRESSION THEORIES

For most people, mood is such a dominant aspect of life. When we are in a great mood, it almost seems like nothing can go wrong, and, if something does, we are able to cope adequately. Unfortunately, when our mood goes sour, just the opposite is true and it appears that nothing can go well. Even seemingly positive events can be stressful when we are in a pessimistic or bad mood. But what happens in the brain to cause a good or bad mood, and how do these chemicals trigger certain behavior? Is it possible that after weeks of feeling low or depressed, a drug can quickly lift your spirit and allow you to function optimally? I will explain all of this to you in the following section.

Neurotransmitters and Mood

Generally speaking, our moods are determined by chemicals in our brains called neurotransmitters. These neurotransmitters act as chemical messengers for neurons, or the gray matter in our brains. Overall, neurons function quite simply, since all they do is receive information and then transmit it to the next neuron. The end of the neuron that receives messages is called the dendrite and is filled with neurotransmitter receptor sites. Neurotransmitters bind to these receptor sites and when enough have been filled, the neuron transmits a signal to its transmission end, the terminal buttons, which, in turn, are filled with neurotransmitters that are released and travel to the next neuron. This process occurs millions of times in different parts of our brains every second and is how information is processed. What makes our brains so complicated is the sheer number of neurons, neurotransmitters, and receptor sites in them. There are hundreds of different neurotransmitters, each one having possibly dozens of different receptor sites that it can bind with, along with billions of neurons. This makes for a massive and complicated information processing system.

Scientists have found that different areas of the brain have specific functions. For instance, while reading this page you are using an area of your brain termed the visual cortex. Neurons pick up information from your eyes and then send it to the visual

cortex at the back of the brain, where the information is processed and sent to other parts of your brain.[1] (Its location is why
people might "see stars" when they hit the back of their
heads.)

There are three main areas of the brain—the hindbrain,
midbrain, and forebrain. The hindbrain and midbrain contain
structures that process body functions like heart rate, breathing,
balance, coordination, muscle movement, and some sensory
information. These types of functions are considered "lower"
brain functions because they're automatic—that is, we don't
have to "think" about doing them. The forebrain processes both
lower brain functions like hunger, thirst, and sensory information, and "higher" brain functions such as memory, logic, con-
scious thought, vision, hearing, and language. Included in the
forebrain is the limbic system, a network of structures that process emotion.[2] The neurotransmitters at work in these areas are
targeted by antidepressants.

The class of neurotransmitters known as monoamines has
been shown to have a major effect on emotion and mood. Three
particular monoamines—noradrenaline (norepinephrine), serotonin, and dopamine—have been heavily researched. All three
of these neurotransmitters are found throughout the body as
well as in the brain and are involved in both brain and bodily
functions. This is why there can be so many side effects to
taking medications like antidepressants that alter the levels of
monoamines. Two monoamines in particular, noradrenaline
and serotonin, have been consistently connected to psychiatric
mood disorders such as depression and bipolar disorder. Another
neurotransmitter, dopamine, the precursor to noradrenaline, is
commonly associated with the pleasure system of the brain.
Disruption to the dopamine system is linked to psychosis and
schizophrenia, a severe mental disorder characterized by distortions in reality and illogical thought patterns and behaviors.

Neurons affected by serotonin are found in almost every
region of the forebrain, including the limbic system. Since sero-

tonin neurons are widespread throughout the body, they are connected to a variety of functions, such as sleep, wakefulness, eating, sexual activity, impulsivity, learning, and memory.[3] Researchers believe that abnormal serotonin levels may lead to abnormal emotional functioning and mood disorders (depression and bipolar disorder). There are a variety of drugs that can affect serotonin levels, which I will discuss in chapter 8.

Noradrenaline neurons are also found throughout the forebrain and related substructures such as the limbic system. Researchers have found that noradrenaline neurons are generally inactive during activities like eating and sleeping but are much more energetic when we are active during the day. It is believed that noradrenaline neurons help to coordinate appropriate responses while we are interacting with the world around us. In contrast to serotonin, which is associated with sleep, depression, and memory, noradrenaline is generally associated with the body's alert and active state.

Depression Theories and Corresponding Medications

Researchers believe that abnormal levels of serotonin and noradrenaline are some of the primary causes of mood disorders such as depression and bipolar disorder. While they do not know the exact process by which levels of serotonin and noradrenaline affect depression, there are several widely held theories.

The *Biogenic Amine Hypothesis* was one of the earliest biological explanations for the cause of depression. In the 1950s, researchers discovered that drugs that decreased monoamine levels (noradrenaline, serotonin, and dopamine) seemed to make patients depressed, while drugs that increased their levels relieved depression. This led researchers to conclude that it was the low levels of monoamines in specific brain regions that caused depression. By this reasoning, depression could be successfully treated with drugs that increase monoamine levels— specifically serotonin and noradrenaline. Dopamine, the

neurotransmitter that affects smooth muscle function, is defi-
cient in individuals with Parkinson's disease, which is why this
disease affects a person's normal movements. Serotonin and noradrenaline are more connected with mood disorders—especially
depression.

One class of drugs that raises the levels of monoamines is
monoamine oxidase inhibitors, or MAOIs. There are dozens of
different MAOIs, but three of the most commonly used include
Nardil (phenelzine), Parnate (tranylcypromine), and Marplan
(isocarboxazid). These drugs work by blocking the action of
monoamine oxidase (MAO) in the nervous system. After monoamine neurotransmitters are released into the synapse (the space
between two neurons), the MAOI medication breaks down some
of the monoamine. Remember that neurons transmit and receive
information by using neurotransmitters. By raising the levels of
monoamines in the synapse, there is a greater chance the message
from one neuron will get to the next neuron. In general, MAOIs
affect all three neurotransmitters—noradrenaline, serotonin, and
dopamine. Since all of these neurotransmitters are responsible for
a wide variety of brain and body functions, altering the levels of
monoamines can also lead to serious side effects.

Another class of drugs that raise neurotransmitter levels is
the reuptake inhibitors. The most common reuptake inhibitors
are targeted at serotonin or noradrenaline and have fewer side
effects than MAOIs. After a neuron releases a neurotransmitter
into the synapse and it binds to a receptor site, some of it will be
recollected by the same neuron that released it. This process is
called reuptake. By blocking this process, reuptake inhibitors
increase the amount of serotonin or noradrenaline in the synapse,
like the MAOIs do but by a different mechanism. This means
that there is a greater chance that messages will get passed from
one neuron to the next. Selective serotonin reuptake inhibitors
(SSRIs) are more commonly used today than noradrenaline-
specific drugs. Prozac (fluoxetine), Paxil (paroxetine hydrochlo-
ride), Zoloft (sertraline), Serzone (nefazodone), Celexa (citalopram

hydrobromide), and Lexapro (escitalopram oxalate) are commonly prescribed SSRI medications. Both Remeron (mirtazapine) and Wellbutrin (bupropion) are inhibitors of noradrenaline and dopamine reuptake with no direct action on serotonin.[4]

While increasing the levels of neurotransmitters in the synapse seems like a process that would immediately improve depression, research has shown that MAOIs and SSRIs often take weeks to fully take effect on major depression. Yet, research has also shown that these drugs increase levels of serotonin and noradrenaline within hours, so there must be some additional process at work that causes depression besides simple neurotransmitter levels. The final explanation for this is still forthcoming, as the scientific studies continue to unfold.

The *Receptor Sensitivity Hypothesis* takes into account the effect of receptor sites on neuron function. The receptor end of a neuron (the dendrite) can have different levels of sensitivity. It is believed that a neuron will synthesize, or create more receptor sites, when neurotransmitter levels are low. This process of creating more receptor sites is called up-regulating and takes weeks to accomplish. When a neuron has an unusually large amount of receptor sites, the neuron is said to be supersensitive. The Receptor Sensitivity Hypothesis says that depression is caused by this supersensitivity and up-regulation. The depression is treated by increasing the levels of neurotransmitters so that the neuron will compensate by reducing the number of receptor sites, a process called down-regulation. Since up- and down-regulation take weeks, antidepressant medications need to be taken on a long-term basis. The length of time needed for neurons to down-regulate may offer one explanation of why antidepressants take up to 6 to 8 weeks to have a full effect on depression.

Another theory that attempts to explain the cause of depression is the *Serotonin Only Hypothesis*. This theory is similar to the Biogenic Amine Hypothesis but states that serotonin, and not noradrenaline, is the principal neurotransmitter involved in depression. This theory gained credibility in the early 1980s with the introduction of the SSRIs. But later studies suggested that both noradrenaline and serotonin working simultaneously may be important in depression and its treatment. Effexor (venlafaxine) appears to work on both systems as does Cymbalta (duloxetine) and both are serotonin-norepinephrine reuptake inhibitors (SNRIs). A more recent theory—the serotonin-norepinephrine-dopamine hypothesis—assesses that all three neurotransmitters may be involved in the biochemistry of depression. Hence several new SNDRIs are now being tested in various phases of pharmaceutical development at Fieve Clinical Services and Sepracor Inc.

Current research supports the *Permissive Hypothesis* of depression, which emphasizes the balance between serotonin and noradrenaline. Research suggests that serotonin helps regulate other neurotransmitters, especially noradrenaline. When serotonin levels fall too low, other neurotransmitters are not as inhibited, and their unregulated effects can impact mood. The Permissive Hypothesis states that depression is caused by the combination of low levels of both serotonin and noradrenaline. Remember that noradrenaline is associated with the brain's more activating functions, such as interacting with the world. If noradrenaline levels are too low, a person may not be very effective in coping with the world around him or her and, in turn, might be depressed. But, if noradrenaline levels are too high and serotonin levels remain low, the person might become hyperactive in relating to the world; this would explain mania and hypomania. Thus, the Permissive Hypothesis can explain the cause of both depression and bipolar disorder. SNRIs such as Cymbalta (duloxetine) work by increasing both serotonin and noradrenaline in hopes of creating a balance of both neurotransmitter hormones.

UNDERSTANDING THE BIPOLAR SPECTRUM

Mood disorders include a large group of psychiatric conditions in which abnormal moods and physical disturbances such as changes in sleep patterns, eating habits, and motion (either speeded up or slowed down) dominate the clinical picture. Known in previous editions of the *DSM* as affective disorders, the term "mood disorders" is preferred by psychiatrists today because it refers to sustained emotional states and not merely to the external mood, or affective expression, of the person's present emotional state. Mood disorders are syndromes (rather than discrete diseases), consisting of a cluster of signs and symptoms that are sustained over a period of weeks to months, and that represent a marked departure from a person's habitual functioning. They tend to recur often in periodic or cyclical fashion.

Though the symptoms of mania and depression were recognized thousands of years ago, it wasn't until the beginning of the 20th century that manic depression was recognized and formally labeled. The term "bipolar" was coined in 1953 by Karl Kleist, MD, a pioneer in German neuropsychiatry. Officially, the term "bipolar disorder" was first used in psychiatry to make a clear division between the two opposite poles: the episodes of elated mood or mania, and the episodes of major depression.

Still, so much myth and misinformation surround bipolar disorder that most people are completely unaware that there is a full spectrum of mood states. While it used to be thought that depression and manic depression were two independent illnesses, we now know that these are two extremes on a continuum with myriad variations found at all points in between. For example, we now believe that full-blown mania represents one extreme, and highly recurrent major depression (without mania) represents the other. Whereas those with Bipolar I may experience mild to major depression along with the psychotic manic highs (the twin poles of their disorder), people afflicted with unipolar major depression experience only the down phase with no mania or highs.

When the high and low episodes happen repeatedly over a course of months or years, we consider the psychiatric illness

Mood Disorders in the Bipolar Spectrum

- Bipolar I mixed states

- Bipolar II disorder

- Bipolar IIB (beneficial)

- Bipolar III (medication-triggered hypomania)

- Schizoaffective (bipolar) disorder

- Cyclothymia

- Hyperthymia

- Hypothymia

- Dysthymia or mild depression

- Chronic major depression

- Rapid-cycling

- Ultra-rapid-cycling[5, 6]

- Unipolar hypomania

to be recurrent. Between these extremes is a range of bipolar conditions (see above).

In addition, there is unipolar hypomania (a mild high without any low mood). Though there is little doubt that it exists, it is difficult to do an epidemiologic study on unipolar hypomanics because they never go to a psychiatrist's private office or a clinic; unipolar hypomania, therefore, is not included as a diagnosis in the *DSM-IV*, nor is Bipolar IIB (beneficial), discussed further in chapter 6.

With all of these varying degrees of bipolar disorder, multiple mood symptoms can often make the diagnosis challenging for a psychiatrist. For example, if a patient has symptoms of psychosis with hallucinations (hearing, seeing, or sensing stimuli that are not present) and delusions (irrational, often paranoid, false beliefs that cannot be explained), a doctor may give the diagnosis of schizophrenia or Bipolar I disorder. Yet the two psychiatric illnesses are quite different. According to the *DSM-IV*, schizophrenia, literally meaning "split mind," is a heartbreaking and disabling brain disease that causes severe mental disturbances and is difficult to manage. Symptoms include delusions, hallucinations, hearing voices that are not there, incoherent speech, and grossly disorganized or catatonic behavior with rigidity or extreme flexibility of the limbs. A person with Bipolar I may suffer with elated mania with or without delusions and psychosis, alternating with major depressive episodes, and then return to a fully functional mood between these mood states. The Bipolar I patient may have periodic hospitalizations, working with a team of mental health specialists who try to find the right combination of medications to stabilize the mood. In extreme unmanageable cases of Bipolar I, electroconvulsive therapy (ECT) is used to try to normalize the body's biochemical mayhem.

To get a better understanding of the bipolar spectrum, let's look at the various mood categories. It is important to note that these categories are simply groupings. Everyone's mood is different, and mood states can fit anywhere on the continuum between these main categories.

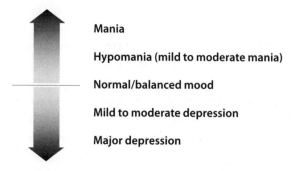

Mania

Hypomania (mild to moderate mania)

Normal/balanced mood

Mild to moderate depression

Major depression

Mania

Mania, the fundamental mood episode that characterizes Bipolar I disorder, is an abnormally persistent, elated, and expansive mood that causes profound morbidity and impaired functioning. With this highly charged but unstable mood state, there are behavioral symptoms such as a decreased need for sleep, physical hyperactivity, euphoria, religiosity, irritability, and even psychosis. Because of the impaired insight and perception, many patients are not compliant with medications, which makes it quite difficult to stabilize the moods.

For Martin, the manic state was terrifying, as his mind took him to a frightening place filled with paranoid delusions and hallucinations. I met this 58-year-old landscape architect and his wife, Camille, last fall at my private practice. Camille revealed to me that Martin had undergone a major depressive episode a few months before when faced with a series of stressful events—the loss of both parents within weeks of each other and then a sudden diagnosis of prostate cancer. While the cancer had been operated on and treated successfully, Martin suddenly began exhibiting strange behavior, staying awake several nights in a row with fears that someone was breaking into their home. Martin would pace the hallway and check each window in the home several times throughout the night. He even installed additional deadbolts and chain locks on their already secure doors. Camille said nothing about this new and questionable behavior until she began to notice that Martin was carrying a small tape recorder in his bathrobe pocket at night. When questioned about it, he became quite agitated and whispered that it was to tape the men's voices he had overheard outside their bedroom window. He wanted to give the police the tapes as evidence in case of a robbery. At first Camille believed her husband's story. Why not? He was a bright, creative professional and had never done anything to make her doubt him. Feeling nervous, she decided to stay up with him to see if people really were outside the bedroom window.

It was midnight, and Camille and Martin were very quiet, listening intently for anyone who might be outside the window. But suddenly, when Martin started to yell at the voices he heard and Camille heard nothing but the neighbor's cat, she realized that something about her husband's perception was not normal. When Martin finally went to sleep at about 3:00 a.m., Camille slipped out of bed, found his tape recorder, and played several of the recordings that he had made. While each tape was carefully documented with the date and time, not one tape had voices on it; they all were blank. The next morning Camille made arrangements with Martin's internist and a psychiatrist to have him admitted to the psychiatric hospital so he could be medically and psychiatrically evaluated. His diagnosis was Bipolar I with psychosis. The attending psychiatrist stabilized Martin's mood with lithium, and he was released a week after the manic episode.

During a full manic episode, the emotional state is highly volatile and often charged with extreme energy and flight of ideas. As Martin experienced, it is not uncommon for a Bipolar I patient with mania to go 2 or 3 days or more without any sleep—and not miss it. In the most severe form of the illness, manic patients become psychotic with hallucinations or delusions, both paranoid and euphoric.

Even though Bipolar I patients use the word "high" to describe their manic episodes, the mood frequently is not euphoric but rather dysphoric or irritable; paranoid with an irrational distrust of others; or angry, leading to panic, confrontations, and rage attacks. In its most severe form, known as psychotic mania, the Bipolar I patient may hear voices and have grandiose delusions such as "I am the new King of England." You've probably read stories about people who thought they heard God speaking to them, or more likely, they thought they were God themselves. Maybe you remember reading about a few Hollywood actors who were caught hiding behind buildings or in the bushes thinking the CIA was after them. While you might recognize that as unusual behavior, most manic patients themselves seldom recognize that they are ill and refuse to see psychiatrists or take medication, blaming everyone around them as "crazy." However, when severe mania is left untreated, the risk of full psychosis and collapse brought on by physical and mental exhaustion greatly intensifies. When Bipolar I mania gets to that point, it becomes difficult to stabilize, is resistant to treatment, and requires hospitalization.

With Bipolar I mania, hospitalization is usually necessary to protect these patients from harming themselves or others. Often, this hospitalization is at the request of the family, and, unfortunately, it must occasionally be legally forced by having two psychiatrists deem that the patient presents a threat to himself or to others in the community.

The *DSM-IV* gives the following criteria for a manic episode:[7]

A. "A distinct period of abnormally and persistently elevated, expansive, or irritable mood, lasting at least 1 week (or any duration if hospitalization is necessary).

B. During the period of mood disturbance, three (or more) of the following symptoms have persisted (four if the mood is only irritable) and have been present to a significant degree:

1) Inflated self-esteem or grandiosity
2) Decreased need for sleep (e.g., feels rested after only 3 hours of sleep)
3) More talkative than usual or pressure to keep talking
4) Flight of ideas or subjective experience that thoughts are racing
5) Distractibility (i.e., attention too easily drawn to unimportant or irrelevant external stimuli)
6) Increase in goal-directed activity (either socially, at work or school, or sexually) or psychomotor (relating to muscles) agitation
7) Excessive involvement in pleasurable activities that have a high potential for painful consequences (e.g., engaging in unrestrained buying sprees, sexual indiscretions, or foolish business investments)

C. The symptoms do not meet criteria for a mixed episode. (Symptoms of a mixed episode include agitation, trouble sleeping, significant change in appetite, psychosis, and suicidal thinking.)

D. The mood disturbance is sufficiently severe to cause marked impairment in occupational functioning or in usual social activities or relationships with others, or to necessitate hospitalization to prevent harm to self or others, or there are psychotic features.

E. The symptoms are not due to the direct physiological effects of a substance (e.g., a drug of abuse, a medication, or other treatments) or a general medical condition (e.g., hyperthyroidism).

Note: Maniclike episodes that are clearly caused by somatic antidepressant treatment (e.g., medication, electroconvulsive therapy, and light therapy) should not count toward a diagnosis of Bipolar I disorder."

Signs of Bipolar I Mania

- Increased energy, activity, restlessness, racing thoughts, and rapid talking
- Excessive "high" or euphoric feelings
- Extreme irritability and distractibility
- Decreased need for sleep
- Unrealistic beliefs in one's abilities and powers (delusions)
- Uncharacteristically poor judgment
- A sustained period of behavior that is different from usual
- Increased sexual drive
- Abuse of drugs, particularly cocaine, alcohol, and sleeping medications
- Provocative, intrusive, or aggressive behavior
- Denial that anything is wrong
- Psychosis and hallucinations

Hypomania

Hypomania, meaning, literally, "mild mania," is an essential mood state that characterizes Bipolar II disorder, along with the occurrence of one or more major depressive episodes. Unlike the mania of Bipolar I, this "mild mania" associated with Bipolar II disorder usually does not impair the person's daily functioning or cause a need for hospitalization. Most patients do not remember past periods of hypomania because they enjoy them immensely, making diagnosis difficult for physicians. In fact, the *DSM-IV* calls for observation and documentation of the hypomania by others (spouses, family members, and friends) in order to confirm the true Bipolar II diagnosis.

When I talk about Bipolar II disorder, especially the hypomanic person with incredible energy, creative ideas, and productivity, many people ask me how a mental illness can be an advantage. Granted, Bipolar I is very difficult to manage with its extreme mania and depression and often lack of compliance to medications and regular doctor's visits. But a person with Bipolar II often thrives on the energizing hypomania and could easily be the CEO of a major corporation, a Wall Street high roller, or a high-ranking government official.

Many patients with Bipolar II find that the hypomanic state greatly enhances their creativity and productivity. Lauren, a 40-year-old graphic artist, described hypomania in the following way:

"Without fail, I can sense the hypomanic state start to take over in early spring. Perhaps it's from the increase in daylight hours or maybe because I spend more time outdoors. I awaken one day after weeks of a low-grade depression, feeling very much focused, alive, and creative. As if overnight, I am transformed into the next van Gogh or Dalí. I long to explore my creativity and I almost dread having to sleep at night, thinking of it as a waste of time. During this period, I drop down to about 3 or 4 hours of sleep at most.

"My paintings are now effortless, and I can finish one in

just hours. The color combinations are like none I've used before with brilliant blues, crimson reds, and shimmering greens that emanate over the entire canvas, giving the painting immense dimension and making the still life appear animated. During this hypermanic state, I also feel exceptionally alert and hypersexual. It is not unusual for me to go out with a different man every night of the week, even when I must be at work by 7:30 the next morning. When I do a gallery showing, I just sense that the world is in love with me and my art. Last year, after showing (and selling!) four of my watercolors, a gallery in lower Manhattan offered to include me in their fall opening."

As Lauren described, with hypomania, the person shows a high level of energy, ideas, creativity, and productivity and may be overactive socially, physically, and sexually. Characteristically tireless, they may be garrulous and expansive, and charming. Those with hypomania are often seductive, wearing flamboyant clothes and exhibiting behavior that may be considered risqué or inappropriate.

Bipolar Depressive and Hypomanic Mood States

DEPRESSION	HYPOMANIA
Tired	Energized
Dull	Alert
Pessimistic	Optimistic
Gloomy	Bright
Hopeless	Hopeful
Feeling of gloom	Excited
Tearful	Laughter
Quiet	Talkative
Empty	Enthusiastic
Withdrawn	Outgoing
Melancholy	Cheerful
Poor concentration	Focused

With Bipolar II hypomania, the person may also have excessive moodiness and impulsive or reckless behavior when she gets too "high." While people with mania have severely impaired function and are out of control (they can hurt themselves and others), hypomania is a milder state in which people are active and productive although highly irritable—but *not* a physical threat to themselves or others unless they exhibit reckless sexual, spending, or driving behavior.

It is sometimes difficult to draw a distinct line between "manic" and "hypomanic," since "marked impairment" versus "little to no impairment" is necessarily a subjective evaluation. In other words, what may be grandiose to one person may be commonplace to someone else. Oftentimes, people who are hypomanic overestimate their own abilities. As the mildly elated mood develops, at times coming dangerously close to mania, individuals may take irresponsible risks, drive recklessly, travel extensively, talk incessantly, or participate in a multitude of sexual liaisons.

One fairly reliable indicator of hypomania is the amount of sleep a person needs. Someone who sleeps just 3 hours a night is usually hypomanic, but he or she may have no complaints about this type of insomnia (in fact, they probably feel refreshed). I have many Bipolar II patients who sleep 3 or 4 hours a night when they are hypomanic, yet increase sleep to 10 or more hours when they are in the depressed phase. Additionally, those with hypomania (and mania) often have "pressured speech," which is a rapid-fire speaking pattern whereby they talk constantly, interrupt, and speak so fast they cannot be understood. In some people with Bipolar II, the pressure of speech usually manifests as extreme outspokenness or persuasiveness—a useful trait in sales, legal careers, evangelism, or politics.

The associated signs of mania (page 45) are present in a much milder form in hypomanic episodes, except that delusions are never present.

According to the *DSM-IV*, the criteria for a hypomanic episode are as follows:[8]

A. "A distinct period of persistently elevated, expansive, or irritable mood, lasting throughout at least 4 days, that is clearly different from the usual nondepressed mood.

B. During the period of mood disturbance, three (or more) of the following symptoms have persisted (four if the mood is only irritable) and have been present to a significant degree:

1) Inflated self-esteem or grandiosity
2) Decreased need for sleep (e.g., feels rested after only 3 hours of sleep)
3) More talkative than usual or pressure to keep talking
4) Flight of ideas or subjective experience that thoughts are racing
5) Distractibility (i.e., attention too easily drawn to unimportant or irrelevant external stimuli)
6) Increase in goal-directed activity (either socially, at work or school, or sexually) or psychomotor agitation
7) Excessive involvement in pleasurable activities that have a high potential for painful consequences (e.g., engaging in unrestrained buying sprees, sexual indiscretions, or foolish business investments)

C. The episode is associated with an unequivocal change in functioning that is uncharacteristic of the person when not symptomatic.

D. The disturbance in mood and the change in functioning are observable by others.

E. The episode is not severe enough to cause marked impairment in social or occupational functioning, or to necessitate hospitalization, and there are no psychotic features.

F. The symptoms are not due to the direct physiological effects of a substance (e.g., a drug of abuse, a medication, or other treatment) or a general medical condition (e.g., hyperthyroidism).

Note: Hypomanic-like episodes that are clearly caused by somatic antidepressant treatment (e.g., medication, electroconvulsive therapy, light therapy) should not count toward a diagnosis of Bipolar II disorder."

Normal/Balanced Mood

With normal mood, the person does not complain of having a mood that is too high or too low, nor do family and friends observe or complain about symptoms or behaviors of extreme mood states.

Mild to Moderate Depression

If you've ever felt completely unmotivated and apathetic for several years on end, along with little appetite, difficulty sleeping, and low-grade fatigue, perhaps you had mild depression (called dysthymia). Forty-three-year-old Elliot had suffered with mild depression off and on since young adulthood. He had tried psychotherapy for a few years but with little or no response. After reading numerous articles on the Internet that described remarkable improvement of depressive symptoms with the newer antidepressant drugs, he called and made an appointment to see me. Elliot reported in the initial interview that for 4 or 5 years, even though he managed to function as an attorney and was happily married with two teenagers, he had not felt like his previous normal self and was only going through the motions of life with very little pleasure, often in a slight daze and in slow motion. After a physical examination and a careful psychiatric evaluation along with a discussion of his family history, I diagnosed him as suffering from chronic dysthymia and started him on the antidepressant Cymbalta. Within 3 weeks, he reported that this drug had made a dramatic difference and changed his mood from chronic pessimism to normal optimism. Elliot said he was enjoying his family more, feeling highly motivated at work, and planning a cruise to celebrate his 20th wedding anniversary. Not only was his energy level back to normal, but he did not feel as if a daily dark cloud was hanging over him anymore.

Dysthymia, a term coined in the 1980s for minor depression, was previously tagged "depressive neurosis" in the 1950s and "depressive personality" in the 1970s. The National Institute of Mental Health estimates that dysthymia affects about 1.5 percent of the US population age 18 and older during their lifetimes, or about 3.3 million American adults.[9] The average age of onset is 31. About 40 percent of adults with dysthymic disorder also meet criteria for major depressive disorder or Bipolar I or II disorder in a given year.[10] While not disabling like major depression, dysthymia generally keeps a sufferer from feeling well and functioning optimally.

According to the *DSM-IV,* a diagnosis of dysthymic disorder[11] includes the following:

A. "Depressed mood for most of the day, for more days than not, as indicated either by subjective account or observation by others, for at least 2 years. Note: In children and adolescents, mood can be irritable and duration must be 1 year.

B. Presence, while depressed, of two (or more) of the following:

1) Poor appetite or overeating
2) Insomnia or hypersomnia
3) Low energy or fatigue
4) Low self-esteem
5) Poor concentration or difficulty making decisions
6) Feelings of hopelessness

C. During the 2-year period (1 year for children or adolescents) of the disturbance, the person has never been without the symptoms in Criteria A and B for more than 2 months at a time."

With dysthymia, it is important that your doctor rule out other problems that may result in similar symptoms, such as substance abuse (particularly marijuana), general medical conditions such as hypothyroidism or anemia, and even certain cancers.

Major Depression

You've probably felt low or sad at some point in your life. Having brief periods of sad feelings often accompanies the usual day-to-day events of life. This type of feeling down or sad can be a normal reaction to disappointing life events or the reaction to a loss, if it is short-lived or transitory. Once the adverse events are resolved, you can adapt to the circumstances, and the feeling of being down usually fades away.

Whether depression is biochemical in origin, or reactive, or a combination of the two, depends on the person and his genetic background and the current situation. Reactive depression is a normal response to a loss; it usually goes away within 1 to 2 months. Its seriousness is in proportion to the impact of the loss, and it most often does not lead to suicide. Major recurrent depression without mania and severe Bipolar I or Bipolar II depression do not act this way. Sometimes patients fail to realize (or accept) that there is a physical cause to their depressed moods and search endlessly for external causes as the reason. The suicide risk in people with biochemical depressions of this nature is the highest seen in any psychiatric state. In fact, it is estimated that by the year 2020, major depression will be second only to ischemic heart disease in terms of the leading causes of morbidity in the world.[12]

Major depressive disorder affects approximately 14.8 million American adults (about 6.7 percent of the US population age 18 and older in a given year). It is a leading cause of disability in the United States and worldwide market economies.[13] The median age of onset of major depressive disorder is 32. Many patients with Bipolar I and Bipolar II experience major depression where they are in a depressed mood most of the day, for weeks or months at a time.

As an example, after experiencing lengthy periods of major depression interspersed with hypomanic episodes, Stephanie, a 31-year-old doctoral student, was diagnosed with Bipolar II disorder a decade ago. She wrote the following during a recent office visit as she described her low mood:

"My real lows began when I went away to college, although I remember having a few shorter periods of depression in high school. I also had a history of bulimia in high school and had secretly been drinking alcohol at night when my parents went to bed or before going out on a date. I remember filling the bottle of vodka with water after I made a few drinks, so my parents would not find out. What I didn't know at the time was that I was really trying to soothe my anxiety and low mood.

"I was awarded a full scholarship to Barnard, but when I started my undergraduate classes, I was petrified. Not only was I extremely anxious about the new situation, but I started feeling panicked and afraid to speak out in class, which had never bothered me before. I was terrified that I would be criticized by the professor or by a classmate. When I was called upon to answer a question, no words would come out and I would burst into tears and literally run from the class to my dorm room.

"At first, I was afraid to sleep alone in my single dorm room. Then I became afraid that I could not get to sleep, and this fear became volcanic, as it built inside of me. Once I fell asleep, I would wake up almost hourly, for fear I'd sleep through my alarm and miss my classes. By my junior year, I had no friends and had not dated anyone. I studied, went to class, and then returned to my dorm room and locked the door. While lying in my bed each night, I could hear my dorm mates in the hallway getting ready for dates or parties, and I wondered what it felt like to laugh, to look forward to something with anticipation instead of absolute dread. My low mood worsened as the year progressed. I spent more time in my room, skipping classes and sleeping all afternoon. I wanted to quit school, but my parents would hear nothing of it.

"I began to feel increasingly anxious, nervous, and my hands would shake when I would pay for my groceries. I was embarrassed at my situation and became a bit paranoid, thinking that other girls pitied me as I was alone all the time. I honestly thought this was my normal young adult mood. I had no idea that I was sick and very depressed. When I went home the summer after my junior year, my parents noticed the dramatic transformation in my mood, which was now extremely low, lifeless, and almost despondent. I had lost weight, down to 96 pounds, and they were extremely worried. They made an appointment with our family doctor, who then referred me to you.

"On the first visit with you, I told you about the weeks of mild elation and little need for sleep during the summers after my freshman and sophomore years. You diagnosed me with Bipolar II disorder and prescribed lithium combined with Wellbutrin. At first it was difficult getting used to taking medication every day, along with the weekly trips to your office. But once my mood was stabilized, I realized that the tiny pills held the key to ending the darkness of major depression.

"It was like a whole new world opened up to me. I started to love learning again, and my senior year in college was, perhaps, the best year of my life. I met my future husband the fall of my senior year, and we got married 2 years later. Since then, I have completed two master's degrees and am now completing my doctoral dissertation at Columbia. My mood is balanced and very stable. I have no extreme lows or highs and attribute that to the fact that I stay on my medications as directed. I have a sense of humor again and laugh easily. Little things that used to get under my skin do not bother me anymore. I am more accepting of others—and of myself—whereas I used to be extremely critical of everyone around me. When I look back at the extreme major depressive episode I had a decade ago, I can hardly believe that I lived through it."

Major depression, often the clinically depressed phase of Bipolar I or II disorder, is usually recurrent with repeated depressive episodes alternating with normal and high periods throughout one's lifetime. The DSM-IV criteria for major depression require that at least five of the following nine symptoms are present during the same period.[14]

1. "Depressed mood most of the day, particularly in the morning
2. Markedly diminished interest or pleasure in almost all activities nearly every day (anhedonia); these can be indicated by subjective account or observations by significant others
3. Significant weight loss or gain (change of more than 5 percent of body weight in a month)
4. Insomnia or hypersomnia (excessive sleeping) almost every day
5. Psychomotor agitation or retardation (restlessness or slowed down)
6. Fatigue or loss of energy almost every day
7. Feelings of worthlessness or guilt almost every day
8. Impaired concentration, indecisiveness
9. Recurring thoughts of death or suicide (not just fearing death)"

With major depression, one of the symptoms must be either depressed mood or loss of interest, and the symptoms should be present daily or for most of the day, or nearly daily for at least 2 weeks. The depressive symptoms must cause clinically significant distress or impairment in functioning, are not due to the direct effects of a substance (e.g., drug abuse or medications) or a medical condition (e.g., hypothyroidism), and do not occur within 2 months of the loss of a loved one.

Patients with Bipolar II disorder have at least one episode of major depression and at least one hypomanic episode, whereas patients with Bipolar I disorder have a history of at least one manic episode, with or without past major depressive episodes. A patient with unipolar depression has major depression only, without hypomania or mania.

Subtypes of Depression

Perhaps you've felt depressed after a family member or close friend died or maybe after moving to a new city far away from those you love. There are other types of depression that can also coexist with the disorder, including the following:

Double depression is a diagnosis that is made when a patient who has been suffering from chronic, long-term mild depression (dysthymia) plummets into an episode of major depression. Some psychiatrists also use this term to refer to a patient who has a reactive depression because of a recent loss along with bipolar depression or unipolar major depression.

Secondary depression can develop in the presence of a previously existing condition, whether it is medical—such as hypothyroidism, stroke, Parkinson's disease, or AIDS—or psychiatric, such as schizophrenia, panic disorder, or bulimia, among others. The key for the diagnostician is to figure out which one came first—the depression or the medical or psychiatric illness. When the depression clearly develops after the other primary medical or psychiatric condition, it is considered secondary.

Chronic treatment-resistant depression is so persistent that it lasts more than a year and so tenacious that it is unaffected by all major classes of antidepressants and other psychopharmacologic drugs and psychotherapies. Once all classes of antidepressants at maximal dosages have been tried and failed, electroconvulsive therapy is often the final treatment of choice by psychopharmacologists for chronic treatment-resistant depression.

Masked depression refers to depression that is hidden behind physical complaints for which no organic cause can be found. The physician's tendency is usually to dismiss these patients as hypochondriacs or to label them as anxious and recklessly prescribe a variety of tranquilizers to calm them down or stimulants to pep them up and get them out of the office as quickly as possible. Because the neurotransmitters serotonin and norepinephrine influence both mood and pain, it's not uncommon for depressed individuals to have physical symptoms such as joint pain, back pain, gastrointestinal problems, sleep disturbances, and appetite changes, accompanied by slowed speech and physical retardation. Many patients compulsively go from doctor to doctor seeking treatment for their physical symptoms when, in fact, they are clinically depressed.[15]

Because masked depression is especially hard to diagnose correctly and treat effectively, it is frustrating for the patient. It is not uncommon for a person with masked depression to go years without a diagnosis as he or she tries to find answers for vague physical symptoms. Freud himself noted that physical complaints can dominate the clinical picture and lead one to believe that the disorder is strictly physical rather than mental. In the worst case, no doctor is able to properly diagnose and treat the patient, the depression is completely missed, and the patient gives up and commits suicide.

I discuss the treatments for depression in chapter 8. After reading this chapter, talk to your doctor to see if medication (or a change in your current medication) might help you have better quality of life.

BIPOLAR II: MOODSWINGS WITH MILD MANIA (HYPOMANIA)

While Bipolar I disorder is easily diagnosed by the defining manic episode, Bipolar II continues to lag in both diagnosis and treatment. For instance, it is not unusual for Bipolar II disorder to be misdiagnosed as major depressive disorder (page 52), because many patients are more likely to recognize the signs of major depression than the symptoms of mild mania. In fact, although the reason is not clear, some findings indicate that patients with Bipolar I disorder may experience depressive symptoms more than 30 percent of the time, while a Bipolar II patient may have depressive symptoms 50 percent of the time. It could be that Bipolar II patients usually call their doctors to treat depression while most enjoy the mildly high state of hypomania and avoid their doctors altogether during this time. I have treated hundreds of Bipolar II patients with major depression who could not remember a hypomanic state until a spouse or family member reminded them during the initial diagnostic evaluation of the time they spent thousands of dollars on a rare carved elephant collection or quit their job on a whim to open a bar in Tahiti.

When a Bipolar II patient experiences hypomania, it is not always a pleasurable high, particularly when behaviors include being hot-tempered or argumentative. Because so many primary care doctors and some psychiatrists don't associate these negative behaviors with hypomania, the patient's diagnosis is missed or often delayed. That's why a thorough understanding of how Bipolar II moodswings manifest is important to both the reader and the medical community.

The *DSM-IV* diagnostic criteria for Bipolar II disorder include the following:[16]

A. "Presence (or history) of one or more major depressive episodes.
B. Presence (or history) of at least one hypomanic episode.
C. There has never been a manic episode or a mixed episode. A mixed episode occurs when there is a manic episode and a major depressive episode nearly every day for at least a 1-week period.
D. The mood symptoms in criteria A and B are not better accounted for by schizoaffective disorder and are not superimposed on schizophrenia, schizophreniform disorder, delusional disorder, or psychotic disorder not otherwise specified.
E. The symptoms cause significant distress or impairment in social, occupational, or other important areas of functioning."

Gender Differences in Clinical Features of Bipolar I and II Disorder

- Onset of bipolar disorder tends to occur later in women than men.
- Women's mood disturbances more often have a seasonal pattern.
- Women experience depressive episodes, mixed mania, and rapid-cycling more often than men.
- Bipolar II disorder, which has predominantly depressive episodes, is more common in women than men.
- Comorbidity of medical and psychiatric disorders is more common in women than men and adversely affects recovery from bipolar disorder more often in women.
- Thyroid disease, migraine, obesity, and anxiety disorders occur more frequently in bipolar women than bipolar men.
- Substance use disorders are more common in men.[17]

BIPOLAR II WITH RAPID-CYCLING

The course of Bipolar II disorder is marked by relapses and remissions. The lows or depressive episodes alternate with the hypomanic states and normal states. Quite often, there are periods—short or long—of complete wellness between the periods of depression and hypomania, and the patients relate that they have no symptoms during these times (although relatives may report differently). When four or more cyclical mood episodes of illness occur within a 12-month period, the person is said to have *Bipolar II disorder with rapid-cycling.* My colleague David Dunner, MD, and I coined the term *rapid-cycling* in the 1970s when we identified a group of our patients at Columbia who did not respond well to lithium therapy, unlike most of our other Bipolar I and Bipolar II patients. These patients typically had four or more cycles of mania and depression in the 12-month interval prior to lithium treatment. This definition was then adopted formally by *DSM-IV* in 1994 and specifically means the occurrence of four or more mood episodes within the preceding year. In severe cases, rapid-cycling can occur even within a 1-day period to 1-week period.

I believe that rapid-cycling Bipolar II disorder presents a significant challenge with respect to treatment as these patients suffer significant depressive episodes and are at high risk for suicide attempts. Although bipolar disorder is equally common in women and men, research indicates that approximately three times as many women as men experience rapid-cycling. Some Bipolar II patients have *ultra-rapid-cycling,* when episodes occur monthly or more frequently; others have *ultradian rapid-cycling,* which means the symptoms cycle more than once a day.

BIPOLAR III: ANTIDEPRESSANT-INDUCED BIPOLAR DISORDER

When the subtle Bipolar II patients tell their doctors only of symptoms of sadness, impending doom, hopelessness, and fatigue, the disorder is frequently misdiagnosed. Neither the doctors nor the patients realize that the "high" times, or hypomania, are as equal a part of the diagnosis as the depression—and most doctors fail to elicit a history of these recurrent periods of expanded mood interspersed with the periods of major depression. Thus, the patient's symptoms are diagnosed as unipolar major depression only and they are prescribed an antidepressant alone (without a mood-stabilizing drug such as lithium or an anticonvulsant). The resulting sudden switch from depression into symptoms of expansive mood or restless agitation and insomnia with racing thoughts is actually antidepressant-induced hypomania, and it usually occurs within the first 2 weeks of starting antidepressant therapy. Some patients—and even physicians—are surprised and pleased at the depressed person's sudden recovery from depression and their mood transformation. Yet this mood transformation is short-lived as it moves into a hypomanic or even a manic episode. This treatment may then trigger rapid-cycling between depression and hypomania (or depression and mania).

Without proper training and an understanding of the genetic link to bipolar disorder, it is almost impossible for any doctor to tell the difference between major clinical depression and the moodswings of Bipolar II disorder. However, once the patient is given *any antidepressant* and an unexpected or sudden hypomanic reaction occurs, the diagnosis becomes what some psychopharmacologists classify as Bipolar III, and the treatment must be stopped immediately.

The phenomenon of an artificially-induced hypomania, caused by an antidepressant, has been repeatedly documented since the advent of Tofranil (imipramine). It has also been frequently reported in the scientific literature with every known antidepressant drug that has been introduced to the market over the last 4 decades.

It is not surprising that a biochemically depressed patient whose depression does not respond well to the "talking cure" might respond very well (dangerously so) to the right biochemical molecules in the form of a well-tested, FDA-approved antidepressant drug. After all, in the carefully controlled clinical trials conducted throughout the United States and Europe in the mid-1980s (including several of my own studies), Prozac had clearly shown its efficacy in treating bipolar depression. The danger was (and continues to be) the bipolar's hypomanic (or manic) reaction to the SSRI. We have since learned that in patients with a bipolar family history, a mood-stabilizing drug should be given along with the antidepressant to keep the patient's mood from escalating too high into a Bipolar III manic state.

TEMPERAMENTS AND BIPOLAR II DISORDER

There are several mood temperaments often associated with Bipolar II disorder. A temperament is a person's usual mood state or disposition that is not episodic or sporadic. For instance, you might always have an optimistic or cheerful temperament or a consistently irritable disposition. Your best friend or colleague might be overly confident and extroverted in most situations. Mood temperaments are hard-wired in each of us and often determine how we react to life's stressors. For example, if you have a hyperthymic temperament, it might help you to enthusiastically face job challenges. If your spouse or friend has a hypothymic temperament, it might cause them to be more restrained in approaching job tasks.

In most cases, the following temperaments do not require treatment unless they affect day-to-day functioning or, perhaps, progress into Bipolar I or II disorder.

Cyclothymic

The cyclothymic temperament is a volatile mood that consistently fluctuates between mild depression and mild elation, yet neither moodswing is severe enough to fulfill the criteria for bipolar disorder or recurrent depressive disorder. Defined by the *DSM-IV* as a chronic, fluctuating mood disturbance involving periods of hypomanic symptoms and numerous periods of mild depressions, cyclothymic temperament can begin early in life. It is often a precursor to bipolar disorder, or it may remain low-grade and chronic throughout one's lifetime. While cyclothymia is equally common in men and women, more women seek medical treatment. There is a 15 to 50 percent risk that the cyclothymic person may subsequently develop Bipolar I or II disorder.

In the mild hypomanic state of cyclothymia, people may be highly creative, energetic, and productive. In the mildly depressed phase, they are agitated and restless and suffer with insomnia. Some experts believe that cyclothymia may be a mild case of Bipolar II.

Hyperthymic

Hyperthymia is a "top of normal" and "upbeat" mood with some occasional spells of mild depression or dysthymia. This essentially normal personality type is energetic, confident, active, and yet sometimes irritable, over-involved, and meddlesome. Those with hyperthymic temperaments may be talkative, full of goals and plans, and extroverted, similar to what used to be called Type A personality.

Many genetic studies, including those undertaken by my own research team at Columbia, show that people who are hyperthymic may come from a bipolar family in which relatives have struggled with depression, bipolar disorder, suicide, gambling, sociopathy, or alcohol or drug abuse. The family tree often has members with hyperthymic (upbeat) or dysthymic (mildly depressed) personalities. Usually the bipolar family includes one or more relatives who have been highly energetic, creative, and accomplished. If these accomplished relatives have no major moodswings, then they are referred to simply as hyperthymic personalities. On average, these are the people who get things done in all walks of life. Sure, they may irritate you sometimes (they are usually pushy), but they are highly productive, meet deadlines, and have superb outcomes.

Hypothymic

The person who has a fairly even "bottom of normal" mood yet sometimes dips into a mild depression is said to have a hypothymic temperament. The hypothymic person is reasonably well adjusted and functioning but low-key and slightly withdrawn. He or she is a follower rather than a leader, smiles infrequently, works efficiently, and is conscientious. It's been my experience that hypothymics are often perfectionists with obsessive-compulsive traits and prefer a more deliberative pace to life. Less social than the highly charged men and women with hyperthymic and cyclothymic dispositions, hypothymics are usually introverted, steady, and generally conservative in decision making. Psychologists have often identified these people as having a Type B personality.

For Those with Bipolar II and Their Family Members

■ Make sure you fully understand the fundamental differences between mania, hypomania, dysthymia, and major depression, as discussed in this chapter, as well as the various mood states and temperaments in between.

■ Read through the *DSM-IV* diagnostic criteria for each mood disorder described in this chapter, so you are more aware of the warning signs of an impending moodswing. If you or a loved one experiences one or more of these signs, call your doctor for a proper diagnosis and effective treatment, if necessary.

■ Talk openly about the different mood disorders and temperaments and how each person in the family falls into one of these categories. Being open about mood states helps increase acceptance.

■ Make a family pact to alert members if their moods change dramatically. If family members notice that the Bipolar II member is exhibiting unusual behavior, remind the person to check his or her mood symptoms and touch base with the specialist.

■ Develop a good relationship with a psychiatrist or psychopharmacologist that allows you to feel confident in calling him or her any time—day or night—if you feel you need extra support and/or medication.

■ If the patient with Bipolar II starts to go too high or too low and refuses medical treatment, family members should meet with the specialist to develop an action plan that calls for openness, support, education, and medical intervention.

CHAPTER 3

MOODSWING AND FAMILY GENETICS

I recognized the signs of Bipolar II disorder in Caroline almost immediately. This 41-year-old mother of three and accomplished violinist had suffered with episodic depression for almost a decade with periodic occurrences of hypomania. During these periods, she slept about 3 hours and then would spend most of the night writing music, practicing violin, and even walking to the local coffee shop to chat with other "hypomanics" at 3:00 a.m.

As I talked with this bright and expressive woman, she revealed that her father, also a performing artist, was hospitalized with psychosis twice—once in 1980 and again in 1983. While she was unsure of the diagnosis, his doctor did prescribe lithium, which was the gold standard for treating bipolar affective disorder at the time. Her father remained on lithium until his death in 1999. Caroline's mother, also deceased, was an alcoholic; an uncle had committed suicide; several family members took medication for depression; and her brother was a recovering drug addict.

Caroline mentioned that her father's mother suffered with depression for years, and two of her own children had attention-deficit/hyperactivity disorder (ADHD) for which they took medication. I was suspicious that the ADHD in the children might be misdiagnosed and instead be an early manifestation of bipolar disorder. This was definitely a strong bipolar family in my book!

WHAT IS THE BIPOLAR FAMILY?

Today's genetic studies give us great insight into the family linkage of bipolar disorder, and a multitude of controlled studies of affectively ill patients and their first-degree relatives have shown that Bipolar II disorder does, in fact, run in families. In this chapter, I will discuss the strong genetic component of Bipolar II disorder. Using this information, you can talk with extended family members and research your ancestry to see if any family members had signs and symptoms of bipolar disorder or other mood disorders that exist in the bipolar spectrum (see chapter 2). For example, if you have relatives with depression, Bipolar I or Bipolar II, anxiety disorders, substance abuse, and/or attention-deficit/hyperactivity disorder (ADHD), among others, there might be an increased risk for you or your loved ones to have Bipolar II.

In one study at Johns Hopkins University School of Medicine in Baltimore, Sylvia G. Simpson, MD, and colleagues interviewed all available first-degree relatives of patients with Bipolar I and Bipolar II disorder and concluded that Bipolar II disorder was the most common affective disorder in the families of both types of patients. The researchers found that 40 percent of the 47 first-degree relatives of the Bipolar II patients also had Bipolar II disorder; 22 percent of the 219 first-degree relatives of the Bipolar I patients had Bipolar II disorder. A fascinating note, however, was that among the patients who had Bipolar II, researchers identified only *one relative* with Bipolar I disorder. Dr. Simpson concluded that Bipolar II is the most prevalent diagnosis of relatives in both Bipolar I and Bipolar II families.[1]

In further study exploring the genetic linkage of Bipolar II, Stanford University psychiatrist Kiki Chang, MD, director of the pediatric bipolar disorders program, and colleagues have established that children who have at least one biological parent with Bipolar I or Bipolar II disorder have an increased likelihood for getting the same. Dr. Chang reported that 51 percent of the bipolar offspring in one study had a psychiatric disorder, most commonly major depression, dysthymia, bipolar disorder, and attention-deficit/hyperactivity disorder (ADHD). I will discuss ADHD further on page 212, but for now it is important to be aware of these groundbreaking findings linking Bipolar II to ADHD and other mood disorders. Interestingly, the bipolar parents in the study who had a childhood history of ADHD were more likely to have children with bipolar disorder—but not ADHD.[2] Along with the genetic link to bipolar disorder, children of a bipolar parent usually have exposure to significant environmental stressors, such as living with a parent who has a tendency toward wide and unpredictable moodswings, alcohol or substance abuse, financial and sexual indiscretions, and even hospitalizations. While not all children of a bipolar parent will develop bipolar disorder, many do progress to an entirely different psychiatric problem, such as ADHD, major depression, or substance abuse.[3]

In other similar studies, researchers have found that first-degree relatives of a person diagnosed with Bipolar I or II disorder are at an increased risk for unipolar depression (major depression only) when compared with first-degree relatives of those with no history of bipolar disorder. Scientific findings also show that the lifetime risk of affective disorders in people with bipolar family members increases, depending on the number of diagnosed relatives.

While the symptoms of major depression and mania are well-documented with Bipolar I disorder, psychiatrists are still assessing the diagnostic reliability of Bipolar II with its varying degrees of hypomania, along with depression. As I stated in chapter 2, there is a spectrum of manifestations in a bipolar family, including depression alone, alcohol abuse, attempted or committed suicide, gambling, sociopathy (antisocial behavior), ADHD, great achievement, and diagnosed Bipolar I or II disorder. While it is puzzling even to the most astute psychiatrists how these various problems are all part of a mood disorder, an awareness of this genetic propensity can help doctors and patients recognize the symptoms and treat serious problems early on before there is needless suffering.

From Chief Judge to Prison Inmate

Most people remember the day in November 1992 when Sol Wachtler, the preeminent chief judge of New York State's highest court, became the unlikeliest inmate in a federal prison. Arrested for extortion and threatening to kidnap his former lover's teenage daughter, 63-year-old Wachtler was later diagnosed with bipolar disorder.

Pawn of an undiagnosed psychiatric illness? Many said yes, in that Wachtler had no control over his elated and mania-induced actions. In an interview with *Psychology Today,* the former heir apparent to the New York governor's mansion described why he didn't seek help for his manic depression before imprisonment:

"My vanity was one of the reasons I didn't seek help for my illness. Here I was, a manic-depressive. I would check into a hotel room under an assumed name and stay there crying for 2 days without pulling the shade up. My wife, who is a clinical social worker, begged me to get help and told me I was destroying myself. But rather than see a psychiatrist, I got prescriptions for Tenuate [a diet pill], Halcion [a sleeping pill], and Pamelor [an antidepressant]—all from different doctors. I took more than 1,400 Tenuate and 280 Halcion in a 4-month period. After a while, my mood swung from profound depression into a manic state, and I started doing these bizarre things. Yet I never saw it happening . . . "[4]

A prominent Long Island attorney and politician, Sol Wachtler was just 38 when appointed to a trial judgeship by Governor Nelson Rockefeller in 1968. In 1984, New York's Governor Mario Cuomo selected Wachtler to serve as chief judge of the New York Court of Appeals. Happily married with extremely successful children and a host of prominent friends, Wachtler appeared to have it all. There were even rumors that he was being considered to fill the Republican ticket for president or vice president in the future—until his house of cards came tumbling down when Wachtler was named trustee for Joy Silverman's trust. Silverman, a wealthy and attractive woman 17 years his junior, was socially prominent and an active Republican fund-raiser. The fiduciary relationship that transformed into a sexual and sordid criminal affair would eventually strip Wachtler of his judicial title in the state of New York.[5]

After breaking off his affair with Ms. Silverman, Wachtler then changed his mind and sought to win her favor again. This time, she was not interested and was involved with someone else. That is when he started the lovesick attempts to force her hand.[6]

Wachtler was diagnosed with manic depression while he was in jail. The psychologist who treated Wachtler asked if he might have bipolar disorder in his family. At first, the former judge denied this. Then, after reviewing his family history, he found out that his grandmother had died of a violent suicide— not of a broken heart as he had been told since childhood. We now know Bipolar II families characteristically have members who have alcoholism, substance abuse, and a higher suicide rate than either families with Bipolar I or unipolar depression. While some tend to romanticize Bipolar II disorder with its hypomania, in reality, many lives and many families are ruined by this increasingly common disease, which can lead to an increased risk of suicide without proper treatment. Fortunately, as I discuss in chapter 8, there are many highly effective treatment modalities for bipolar disorder.

Family Records Confirm Bipolar

Actress Jane Fonda revealed a similar secret that was well kept in her family's closet in her autobiography *My Life So Far*. Fonda found out that her mother had suffered from manic depression, which drove her to commit suicide when Fonda was 12. In researching family medical records while writing her book, Fonda realized that undiagnosed depression ran deep on both sides of her family and helped explain the moodswings that plagued both her mother and father.

Many times the average practitioner, the public, and those men and women who have symptoms of Bipolar II do not realize the various ways this mood disorder can manifest in people. Sometimes patients and their families hesitate to seek treatment for fear of the "stigma" of having a psychiatric illness, especially if there is a family history of suicide, alcoholism, or substance abuse among relatives. I remember treating a well-known 30-year-old actress in New York who always came to my office under an assumed name and dressed incognito with a black trench coat, dark glasses, and heavy scarf. After learning about her lengthy family medical history filled with major depression, alcoholism, and high achievement, I explained to her that the chances were great that most of her family members had the same disorder. Because of this woman's hypomanic advantage and superb achievements, I diagnosed her with Bipolar IIB (beneficial). She chose to ride out the mild depression with psychotherapy but without medication so she could continue to benefit from the hypomanic periods that boosted her to the top of her field.

Lack of Treatment Can Lead to Suicide

Have you ever been hesitant to openly discuss physical symptoms with your doctor? Many people with bipolar disorder are afraid to discuss their symptoms with their family, friends, and even their physicians. Yet a serious problem arises when signs and feelings are not openly discussed. Not only is the course of Bipolar II disorder distinctly different from Bipolar I or major depression in rates of recovery, clinical features, and number of episodes, but the risk of suicide in Bipolar II is particularly elevated.

The Bipolar II patient often fails to recognize that he or she has a highly treatable depression. This person hesitates to see a psychiatrist for an accurate diagnosis and treatment, preferring to "ride out" the depression. Those with Bipolar II who do seek medical treatment often stop the prescribed medications within weeks or when they feel "well," only to relapse into a deep depression soon thereafter. Bipolar II patients often have a history of suicide attempts or ideation, comorbid substance abuse and/or personality disorders, insomnia, impulsiveness, and family history of suicide. In fact, in a study I published with colleagues at Columbia, we concluded that without effective treatment, Bipolar II disorder could lead to suicide in nearly one out of five cases.[7] Conversely, and it may seem surprising, Bipolar I with episodes of mania is least associated with suicide.

Exploring Family Heritage

Kent is a 32-year-old senior editor of a well-known finance magazine. After reading an interview I did on Bipolar II, he made an appointment to see me. When I met with Kent, I was impressed with how in sync he was with his physical and mental health. He said he had noticed some different feelings over the past few months and described a host of symptoms such as feeling hyperalert all day when normally he would be drowsy and unproductive during the afternoon. Kent told me that he never had problems sleeping at night previously. However, now he was getting a total of 4, maybe 5 hours sleep at night, and he did not miss the sleep. In fact, he said he had started freelance writing for several national publications at night because his mind would not stop its creative flow. As Kent told me, "Mentally, I feel like I'm in a race against time. Even in the wee hours of the morning, my thoughts keep going with no end in sight. The sounds and sights around me are more vivid. I feel like I used to live in black and white and now everything is bright and in full color. I feel very much alive."

Kent and I talked at length about these new feelings. Most definitely he was experiencing feelings of expansiveness—a sign of hypomania. And his oversensitivity to any kind of sound, called hyperacusis, was also an indication of a change in his perception. Kent said he was not taking any medications, nor did he drink alcohol or use recreational drugs. I then asked him if he had any family members who were diagnosed with bipolar disorder, and a flood of information poured forth. Kent was well-prepared for our meeting by knowing his family history and started by telling me about his father, a retired professor, who had never been "diagnosed" with a mental illness that Kent knew of, but who had very quirky habits that always coincided with the change of seasons. Like clockwork, every spring (see "Seasonal Patterns" on page 100) his father would become hyperalert, extremely active, and very religious, which was odd as he was not normally a religious man. While this went on during Kent's teenage years, he didn't pay attention to it. Now, as an adult, when Kent visited during April, his father, almost 80, would talk nonstop, make frequent plays on words, and create clever rhymes and songs that related to what he was doing. He also played religious music all day and well into the night until he fell asleep. This behavior would go on for weeks until early summer, when his father would calm down and be in a more "normal" mood as fall approached. Subsequently, in the fall, when Kent visited his boyhood home, his father would be in slow motion, as if it took all the effort in the world to move his body or talk or even think. When Kent visited his father the previous October, the elderly man did not wake up until almost noon. His speech was slow and almost monotone, and he napped much of the afternoon. While Kent always thought this "contrast" of personality was unusual, his siblings accepted it as part of the aging process.

Kent told me about one spring when he was in college, and his father had lost his job at the university because of budget cuts. While the family was devastated, his father apparently handled the loss and focused on writing a novel. Then on a Saturday night in 1992, Kent's mother called him because his dad was exhibiting "strange" behavior with confusion, agitation at night, and chaotic thinking. She said his dad was keyed up and pacing during the daytime hours, and then stayed awake most of the night, peering out the living room window and whispering about how people from the university were hiding behind the bushes. He was also showing other odd signs of paranoia, such as following behind Kent's mother during the day, as if he did not trust her, and emptying out the garbage in the kitchen, as if he were searching for something but could never find it. When his mother had gone to the grocery store, she said his father had accused her of plotting with the university officials and telling lies about him. After Kent's dad had several nights of little sleep, a police officer in the area found him walking the neighborhood at 4:00 a.m. His father was admitted to the psych ward at the local hospital and stayed there for 2 weeks undergoing tests and evaluations. I asked Kent about the diagnosis, but he said at the time he was so busy with his fraternity and classes, he had no idea what the doctors had said, and his mother had died a few years later. At the time, he excused his dad's behavior as being a result of losing his job at the university. bipolar disorder? Kent had never heard of it until recently.

It's difficult to give a definite diagnosis from secondhand information, but it seemed to me as if Kent's father most likely had Bipolar I disorder, which is characterized by signs of mania with poor judgment, paranoia, and even possible psychosis. His father had also experienced low periods that were consistent with depression. Perhaps the extreme stress of the job loss triggered the manic episode, or maybe it had been happening to a lesser degree before this loss.

After listening to Kent describe his father, I asked about other family members. Were there suicides, relatives with depression or alcoholism, anyone with high achievements? As his family history unfolded before me, I noted that it was a textbook case for a bipolar spectrum family. Over several generations, his family history was marked by both high achievement and psychiatric illness. His older sister, a Harvard-trained scientist and PhD, worked at the National Institutes of Health. I recognized her name immediately and remembered reading of her groundbreaking work on post-traumatic stress disorder (PTSD) and anxiety. His younger sister, an actress in California, never finished high school and had taken Prozac for depression since he could remember. Kent said his grandfather (on his father's side) committed suicide when Kent was 9 years old, but his family was very secretive about it and would not broach the subject with him. Kent remembered that his father's youngest brother, well educated at an Ivy League school, was a staunch member of Alcoholics Anonymous after decades of heavy drinking, bankruptcy, and four failed marriages. His other uncle was a renowned surgeon in Boston, who also had an alcohol problem and had been married three times. This uncle had two sons who were heavy into cocaine. It appeared to me that Kent was genetically predestined to have some type of disorder on this bipolar spectrum.

In my genetic research at Columbia and the New York State Psychiatric Institute, I found numerous epidemiologic studies that substantiated my own findings that members of bipolar families are at increased risk for recurrent unipolar depression, bipolar depression, and schizoaffective disorders, a psychiatric diagnosis where symptoms of both a mood disorder and either psychosis, delusions, or hallucinations are present. The familial genes that are responsible may occur in dissimilar combinations in different relatives. Thus, whereas one family member, like Kent, might have a highly adaptive, high-energy hypomanic mood and be a highly productive Bipolar IIB (beneficial) individual, another family member, like Kent's younger sister, may suffer recurrent bouts of unipolar depression.

When Kent came to me, he said that lately he had been overly "happy," even annoying his wife and co-workers, but he could not control his behavior. At times, he spoke loudly and laughed inappropriately. He walked fast and felt "pumped up" most of the time but had eliminated caffeine and other stimulants from his diet—so it seemed to Kent that the feeling was his natural self. In addition, he had taken to stock trading while sitting at his desk at work. So far, he had made more than he lost, but it still made Kent nervous when he was normally such a calm and conservative rule-follower. "I just want to make sure nothing really serious is wrong," he told me. Then he added, "My wife and I are talking about starting a family, and I want to make sure my genes aren't tainted in any way."

I applauded Kent for being aware of his psychological state. As I noted in the previous chapters, it's not unusual for people with Bipolar II disorder to seek treatment only when a family member or friend has literally dragged them into my office after their mood has extended too high. Sometimes, the person with Bipolar II has run up huge credit card debt or invested a lot of money and lost it all, and the spouse or family member then issues a final ultimatum: "Get a diagnosis and treatment or leave!"

Most people won't discuss Uncle Sid's suicide or Aunt Martha pacing the house at all hours of the night unable to sleep because of "voices she had heard." They shun talking about their own periods of sadness or depression, believing this to be a sign of failure to stand strong and manage their own moods. But I cannot stress enough that the best way to manage moodswings and prevent problems associated with bipolar disorder is to know your family history and discuss it thoroughly with a clinical psychiatrist or psychopharmacologist. Many patients are embarrassed to discuss their history—or their own symptoms. Because some patients are highly successful, they feel the depression period is a sign of "failure." Depression is *not* a sign of failure—it is a treatable problem. A psychiatrist can help the patient put together the pieces of a bipolar family puzzle and prescribe effective treatment, if necessary.

Admittedly, most patients I see spend years living with "mood misery" as they wonder what is happening in their minds but are too afraid to talk to a professional to seek a diagnosis and treatment. I commended Kent for observing his own mood-swings and for the broader awareness of his family history. Hearing the details of his relatives' mood disorders helped me to confidently diagnose Kent with Bipolar II. After a lengthy discussion, Kent agreed to take a small dose of a mood stabilizer to help calm down the hypomania so he could function better at work and in his relationships. He also agreed to monitor his lifestyle and sleep habits and to call me if he found that he was having difficulty sleeping. I could easily prescribe medication and/or therapy to help get Kent back on track before a mood episode flared.

A few weeks after our appointment, Kent and his wife met with a genetic counselor at Columbia Presbyterian Medical Center and felt very positive about the counseling sessions—to the point that his wife is now pregnant. I believe that, by openly discussing his signs and symptoms before he had a serious problem, Kent brilliantly handled his mood disorder, working to make Bipolar II "fit" into his life rather than letting the Bipolar II disorder run—*or ruin*—it.

Diverse Paths

As well as watching for signs of manic depression in your children, it's important to be aware of other related inherited disorders I've discussed in this chapter. I remember a family where I treated one of the daughters for several years for substance abuse and depression. In taking the family history, I was told that her mother was Bipolar I and also an alcoholic with many arrests, including four DUIs. The mother had left the family when the children were ages 2, 4, and 5 (and later committed suicide), so the children grew up without the influence of her next moods. The father, who had no history of psychiatric illness, raised them alone. Even though the three children grew up in the same environment, the younger children (both girls) ran away from home as teenagers, abused drugs for years, were sexually active with many partners at a young age, and dropped out of college after one semester. The oldest son's path was astonishingly different; he made straight A's in honors classes and then went to an Ivy League college on a full scholarship.

Intrigued by the predictability of a bipolar family, I tracked this family for more than a decade. Now in their late twenties, the two sisters who dropped out of college are still struggling to survive without any higher education or training. One continues her addiction to drugs; the other is still an alcoholic, unemployed, and lives alone. As is predictable in a bipolar family, one sibling, the eldest, remained on the path of high achievement and super accomplishments. Now married with two children, he is a board-certified internist in Chicago. His youngest child was just diagnosed with attention-deficit/hyperactivity disorder (ADHD), which we frequently see in bipolar families. While some wonder how three siblings can take such diverse paths, their story confirms the diverse nature of this psychiatric illness in a family.

Success Attributed to Bipolar II

Hugh, a successful salesperson who had risen to the top of his company's sales force at an early age, also came from a bipolar family. Hugh was extremely innovative and dynamic, a consummate negotiator, and a risk taker. He exuded confidence with his lofty mood, high energy, and smooth talk. But when he came to my office, he was suffering with feelings of guilt, despair, and melancholy, yet barely admitting to having a low-grade depression. Hugh said he didn't want to socialize or date, and he was at risk of losing his high-paying job because he could not meet his sales quota. As many with bipolar do, he had complicated his depression by self-medicating with alcohol to assuage his anxiety and stimulant drugs to boost himself up and get out of the depression. He said he even used cocaine frequently. I asked Hugh if he had noticed any periods of hypomania or extreme energy and elation, but he felt so depressed that he could not think of any.

After the psychiatric interview, it was clear to me that this young man had bipolar disorder, probably Bipolar IIB. He had a history of mild, chronic highs interspersed with lows, and he had been able to capitalize on his periods of hypomanic energy to quickly rise to the top of his field.

When I questioned Hugh about his family history, his bipolar story began to unfold. He revealed an aunt who had had severe depressions all her life and who would have probably been diagnosed as having a recurrent major depressive disorder. Two of his sisters appeared to have dysthymia, a form of mild depression lasting a year or more and in which the individual functions normally but below par. His mother had a history of "going to bed for 2 months at a stretch," and he was told that she was "always very tired." Hugh added that one uncle had committed suicide.

I explained to Hugh how family history is crucial in making a proper diagnosis. Bipolar families like Hugh's have a high frequency of both completed suicides and suicide attempts. It is my professional view that if the family histories of these suicidal depressives were fully known by the patient and, thereafter, elicited by the doctor at the initial consultation, we would frequently find in their family heritage many instances of bipolar mood disorder. Although it may help certain people like Hugh to rise to the top of their careers, bipolar disorder can also bring them (and sometimes their family members) down into despair.

Awakened by our discussion of the various moods in his bipolar family, Hugh agreed that he had noticed the signs and symptoms in himself of both depression and hypomania for several years. He made a commitment to take a mood-stabilizing medication and see my practice psychologist regularly to gain an understanding of his mood disorder. He also agreed to join Alcoholics Anonymous and stop taking illegal drugs to calm or stimulate his mood.

Today Hugh continues to do extremely well on lithium and has had no major mood episodes for the past 4 years. He did suffer with a few weeks of mild depression a year ago, but this low mood lifted after adding an antidepressant to the mood stabilizer. Once again, Hugh is at the top of his game in sales, and the long-term outlook for his life and success is excellent.

GENETIC STUDIES REVEAL THE BIPOLAR SPECTRUM IN FAMILIES

I hope I've conveyed how bipolar disorder can result in tremendous human suffering and disrupted lives. But when misdiagnosed, it can result in inappropriate medication, increased health care costs, and a much poorer prognosis, even suicide. Realizing the tremendous health implications of identifying genes that produce vulnerability to mental disorders, researchers have pored over studies, probing for a familial link to age of onset, familial phenotypes, and overlapping bipolar and schizophrenia disorder findings.

By studying families, identical and fraternal twins and their families, and biological families compared to adoptive families, researchers can estimate how genes and environment interplay

to influence bipolar disorder. While no gene has yet been con-
clusively identified, the findings are extremely encouraging.

In the 1960s, after it was first accepted that the two forms
of depression (manic depression and recurrent depression) were
separate illnesses, I started my own genetic studies. From 1972
to 1978, I was a primary author on a number of genetic family
studies conducted on manic depression at the New York State
Psychiatric Institute. The family and genetic linkage studies of
my team, including Julian Mendlewitz, MD, and Joseph Fleiss,
MD, along with studies of others from around the country,
were summed up in the book *Genetic Research and Psychiatry*,
which I edited with colleagues David Rosenthal, MD, and
Henry Brill, MD. At the time, the popular theory was that the
gene(s) controlling for manic depression were located on the X
chromosome and transmitted from mother to son and daughter
or father to daughter, but not father to son. Years later, this
theory was ruled out when we discovered several instances of
male-to-male transmission of the disorder. This large study is a
classic example of the self-corrective process in science, which
means that studies must be replicated in three or four other
laboratories whereby the data published is subjected to peer
review. As it stood, other laboratories across the nation did not
fully replicate our positive X linkage studies in manic depression. Thus, the hypothesis of manic depression being genetically transmitted as a purely X link chromosome disorder has
remained in question.

The importance of these earlier genetic familial studies was
that in my large university clinic, the unprecedented number of
patients and their relatives enabled us to see the many facets of
bipolar disorder and the many forms that it takes in different
people, as I have discussed in this book. Previously, we knew
that children of those with bipolar disorder had a greater risk of
getting the disorder than the general population. However, our
studies in the 1970s and those from other laboratories indicated
that these children were also at risk for a host of *other* problems

later in life that fall into the bipolar spectrum, including drug abuse and alcoholism, suicidal tendencies, and a range of interpersonal difficulties and personality disorders that may mask the underlying disorder.

Knowing the family history is important so we can watch for early behavioral and biochemical clues that one day may allow us to effectively treat the disease much earlier in the afflicted person's life and prevent the adult expression of the disease. Since the late 1990s, cross-sectional studies have reported that about 50 percent of bipolar offspring meet the criteria for at least one *DSM-IV* psychiatric disorder.[8] Nevertheless, when doctors can act early on what we believe are first indications that the child has inherited bipolar disorder or another psychiatric disorder, we are often able to prevent a lifetime of misery caused by what is essentially a highly treatable illness.

Human Genetics Program Uncovers Mysteries

Since the groundbreaking studies on family genetics in the 1970s, so much more has been done to uncover the mysteries of bipolar disorder. In 1989, Elliot Gershon, MD, at the National Institute of Mental Health (NIMH), launched a broad and multifaceted human genetics program for research on very large, three- to four-generation families containing multiple affected individuals. The goal of the initiative was to set up a data bank for use in linking genetic and clinical information for research. In turn, this genetic information would be available for distribution to scientific investigators in the nation. Since that time, researchers have focused on various subtypes of bipolar disorder and have found some intriguing links. For example, most individuals with seasonal affective disorder (SAD), discussed on page 100, also have Bipolar I or Bipolar II disorder. Genes influence the seasonal variation in mood, and seasonal affective disorder appears to aggregate in families.[9] Studies also show there may be a genetic predisposition to rapid-cycling, cyclothymia (see page 62), and unstable moods of borderline personality. Rapid switching of mood may be central to all of these problems and is associated with a more complex course of bipolar disorder. Researchers also believe that eating disorders, impulse control problems, and anxious sensitive personalities run strong in Bipolar II families.[10]

Studies Test the Theory of Nature versus Nurture

Simply because there is a genetic predisposition to bipolar disorder does not mean it will manifest in all members of a family. As with asthma, hypertension, or diabetes, a genetic tendency simply means that the person is more vulnerable to getting the ailment than someone without this inherited susceptibility. There are studies of identical twins (who share the same genes) that indicate other factors in addition to genes play a role in bipolar disorder. If bipolar disorder is caused entirely by genes, then the identical twin of someone with the illness would *always* develop the illness, and research has shown that this is certainly not the case. But we do know that if one identical twin has bipolar disorder, the other twin is more likely to develop the illness than is another sibling.[11]

Environmental stressors also play a role in triggering bipolar episodes in those who are genetically predisposed. Children growing up in bipolar families often live with a parent who lacks control of moods or emotions. Some children may live with constant verbal or even physical abuse if their bipolar parent is not taking medication for the illness or is trying to self-medicate the moodswings with alcohol or drugs.

Genetic Counseling

When I counsel patients with bipolar disorder who are concerned about getting married and having children, I reassure them that by the time the child shows signs and symptoms of bipolar disorder (if he or she ever does), newer treatments even better than lithium or the currently used mood stabilizers may be available. While bipolar disorder has a strong genetic component, early awareness and intervention may help prevent its serious progression in children. With proper education, bipolar parents can watch for early psychiatric difficulties in their offspring and seek professional help early on before the disease leads to out-of-control moodswings or other comorbid behaviors. Genetic research may one day provide us with diagnostic tools and specialized laboratory tests that allow early intervention in children even before the symptoms begin, which I discuss in chapter 9.

Pharmacogenetics and Bipolar II Disorder

Bipolar mood disorder is primarily biochemical and genetic in origin, and there is no other "primary" reason for it. Environment and major stressors, however, may trip off the complex genetic vulnerability and biochemical mechanisms that are responsible for the moodswing. In that light, the *DSM-V*, which will be published in 2012 (tentative date), may be vastly different from the previous four editions, as it will focus more on basing a patient's diagnosis on biological and genetic characteristics. In the fifth edition, the wealth of data from the Human Genome Project (see page 81) will be presented, and researchers will discuss findings on the relationship of many comorbid disorders that appear to run in bipolar families, including ADHD and bipolar disorder, generalized anxiety disorder and bipolar, and unipolar depression and bipolar, among others. In doing so, those in the field of pharmacogenetics, which studies genetic variations in drug response, could play an ultimate role in finding the safest and most effective treatments for specific subtypes of bipolar illnesses.

Numerous family and twin studies now point to genetic

factors as being mainly responsible for variations in how a drug is metabolized and eliminated from the human body. For example, if a Bipolar II patient has a parent or sibling who also has Bipolar II and who has been helped by a certain medication, this same medication may also be the most effective treatment for the Bipolar II patient because of the genetic response. This finding has incredible significance for the psychopharmacologist who seeks to optimize medication effectiveness and prevent drug toxicity in the patient. The physician must consider how quickly a drug will clear the body among different patients before confidently prescribing it, and reviewing a patient's family history of illness and medication may solve the puzzle. I have repeatedly seen that someone with a fast metabolism may require larger or more frequent doses to achieve adequate results while another patient who has a slow metabolism may need much lower doses of a medication or less frequent dosing to avoid toxicity in the body. Once more is known about the patient and his or her genetic makeup for disease and reaction to medication, including how fast a drug is metabolized, absorbed, and eliminated, the prescribing physician may be able to quickly find the most effective drug because of the genetic history.

We continue to be extremely hopeful for a cure for bipolar disorder in the near future. As scientists unravel more about the genetic link of this mood disorder, perhaps the cure will be as clear-cut as introducing a gene into the diseased cell. Until that groundbreaking time, we must find the safest treatments that allow Bipolar II patients to have the greatest quality of life with the fewest side effects.

For Those with Bipolar II and Their Family Members

■ Continue to talk with your immediate family members and extended family about Bipolar II disorder and the associated moodswings. Write down the various diagnoses your relatives have been given, so you can share this information with your physician. By fully understanding your genetic link to bipolar disorder and discussing this with your physician, you can help the doctor prescribe appropriate medication. Without knowing your family history, it is most difficult for a doctor to tell the difference between major clinical depression and the moodswings of Bipolar II disorder.

■ While interviewing different family members, ask about medications they are taking or have taken in the past. What reactions did they have to these medications? Which drugs were most effective or ineffective? Share this information with your physician. These facts may help to solve the mystery behind your mood disorder and medication response and allow you to receive the highest quality of care. You might find that the medication a family member has used is also the best one for you.

■ If you normally feel energetic and productive and are highly successful, don't see the moodswing into depression as a sign of "failure." Depression is a highly treatable problem and part of this mood disorder. Talk to your specialist about the best treatment in your situation.

CHAPTER 4

SLEEP AND BIOLOGICAL RHYTHMS

Judith, a 38-year-old Manhattan real estate broker, told me she rarely felt tired. "Over the past 5 years, I usually got to my office before 7:00 a.m. and stayed until 8:00 p.m. or even later. Then I would meet with clients for drinks or dinner and usually not get back to the apartment until well after midnight.

"On weekends, I was with clients literally all day, showing different properties and closing deals. During a free moment, I'd literally jog to the 92nd Street Y to catch an aerobics class to make up for exercise time I had missed during the week," she said, adding that though she slept only 4 or 5 hours a night, she never napped.

Judith appeared to be the classic success story. After getting a master's in English literature at New York University, she was offered a job at a well-known publishing house, starting as an assistant copy editor and then moving up to an acquisitions editor. However, after a decade of editing for hours each day in her tiny cubicle, Judith told me that all she *gained* was weight— 25 pounds to be exact.

"I was tired of being told what my salary would be each year, no matter how many hours I worked or how successful the book was. I wanted the freedom to be my own boss and set higher financial goals. So, with a close friend, I started a real estate agency, and in less than 3 years, I was making seven figures easily and was called the 'million dollar realtor.'

"The more deals I closed, the harder I worked," Judith said. "It was as if making a substantial property sale was equivalent to a drug addict's fix, and I craved all the fame, power, and money I could get."

Then, over a 1-week period, Judith said that she was working on a megadeal and had a great deal of anxiety; her normal 3 to 4 hours of sleep dwindled to less than 2 hours a night of fitful slumber. Her behavior became unusually elevated, and while normally outgoing, Judith now had racing thoughts and was talking nonstop about the new real estate opportunity to anyone who would listen. During this time, she made several risky deals and appraisals that bordered on not being legal. When her business partner found out, he quickly pulled the company out of two of the more dangerous deals and confronted Judith. It was obvious to her partner that something was very wrong, but Judith denied feeling different. Besides, she liked the invincible, energized, and overly confident feeling she had with the heightened hypomania.

During our first consultation, I diagnosed Judith with Bipolar II disorder. The mild elation that fueled her million dollar sales prowess was out of control, but a combination of therapy and mood-stabilizing medications modulated the hypomania within several weeks.

Two years later, Judith continues to stay on a low dose of a mood-stabilizing drug and an antidepressant and comes to my office monthly for monitoring of blood, medication side effects, and moods. Once again, she is at the top in sales—but now with some modifications in lifestyle, particularly in allowing ample time to relax before she goes to bed. She now has regular office hours that start at 9:00 a.m. and end at 6:00 p.m. If she goes out with clients or friends after work, she makes a point of getting home by 10:00 p.m., so she can do yoga to help her relax and fall asleep. Judith has been told to call me if she notices any change in her sleep habits, so we can find the right combination of medications and therapy before the reduced amount of sleep triggers hypomania.

Now that you have a greater awareness of Bipolar I with its mania and Bipolar II with its hypomania and the genetic component of both types of bipolar disorder, I want to share information on how sleep influences your mood.

I became aware of how little patients with mania actually sleep in the 1960s when I was in charge of the acute psychiatric service at the New York State Psychiatric Institute at Columbia Presbyterian Medical Center. The highly charged men and women I saw lived in a constant agitated and nervous state, even after staying awake for two or three nights at a time, until the manic episode was calmed with ECT or a major tranquilizer. After treating patients with Bipolar I and Bipolar II disorder for years, I realize that disturbances in sleep such as this often give powerful clues in helping to diagnose the abnormal mood states of major depression, mania, and hypomania.

GOOD SLEEP, BAD SLEEP, NO SLEEP

Some findings indicate that individuals with bipolar disorder have a genetic predisposition to sleep-wake cycle abnormalities that may be responsible for triggering the symptomatic manifestations (hypomania, mania, and depression) of the illness.[1] We know that a profoundly decreased need for sleep without noticeable fatigue is consistent with the Bipolar II hypomanic state. While insomnia, or the inability to sleep, does affect 85 percent of those with major depression, these patients usually desire more sleep and do not feel refreshed upon awakening. There are also those individuals in the Bipolar II depressed state who suffer from an irrepressible need to sleep (hypersomnia) and find it difficult to stay awake during daytime hours. After sleeping for 10 to 12 hours, these patients still feel fatigued and lethargic.

Even without any medical or mental health problems, the average American adult gets only an average of 6.9 hours of sleep each night, according to the National Sleep Foundation. (Most experts agree that all adults need between 7 and 9 hours of sleep a night.) About one-third of the adult population suffers with insomnia, the most common sleep disorder in the United States, at some point in their lives. The prevalence of insomnia increases with age and is more common in women than in men. While sleep disturbances often coexist with psychiatric disorders, insomnia without a perceived need for more sleep upon waking from a shortened sleep interval is not observed in any disorder other than bipolar.

The problem for those with bipolar disorder, however, is that sleep loss may precipitate a mood episode of hypomania, or mania in some patients. Worrying about losing sleep can add to cognitive arousal and high anxiety and worsen the psychiatric problem altogether. Once a sleep-deprived person goes into the hypomanic or manic state, the need for sleep is felt even less than before.

Ellen Frank, PhD, director of the depression and manic depression prevention program at Western Psychiatric Institute and Clinic in Pittsburgh, and her colleagues have done tremendous research in the area of sleep and bipolar disorder. In one study, Dr. Frank and her team interviewed 39 bipolar patients with primarily manic or depressed episodes to determine the presence of social rhythm disruptions during the 2 months prior to the onset of the mood. (A social rhythm disruption is a disturbance in routine that affects the sleep-wake cycle.) When comparing the results with those volunteers in the control group, Dr. Frank concluded that most individuals with bipolar disorder experienced at least one social rhythm disruption prior to the mood episode. In addition, the researchers found that social rhythm disruption affected more bipolar patients with mania than the patients with depression. Their findings concluded that 65 percent of the patients with bipolar disorder had at least one disruption in their daily rhythm in the 8 weeks before the onset of a manic episode.[2]

To compare the data, Dr. Frank and her team also looked at the study participants' life events that did not precipitate a manic event during an 8-week period earlier in the year. The researchers rated the life events for both periods. They concluded that the strongest variable in predicting who would experience a bipolar mood episode was *reduction in sleep*. For reasons not yet understood, we think that individuals with bipolar disorder have a more delicate internal clock mechanism, or circadian rhythm. When a social rhythm disruption occurs, such as staying up all night with a sick family member or going to bed late after an evening of partying with friends, it may be enough to trigger hypomania or mania. The researchers are still reviewing whether a social rhythm disruption triggers other events of bipolar disorder such as depression or rapid-cycling episodes.

NORMAL AND ABNORMAL SLEEP

Interest in unraveling the mysteries of sleep has been ongoing since the beginning of time. In 1300 BC, opium was a popular "hypnotic medication" used to treat insomnia in ancient Egypt.[3] In 400 BC, Hippocrates wrote about sleep in the *Hippocratic Corpus,* a library of 34 scholarly books written in the 6th and 4th centuries BC. In the 19th century, there were many sleep theories, including a concept that sleep was related to pressure of blood in the brain (or lack thereof). This idea progressed into behavioral theories, such as the inhibitory reflex, meaning sleep comes about because of something being turned off or removed. The inhibitory reflex theory was then refuted at the turn of the 20th century, when researchers determined that the brain stem played a key role in sleep and wakefulness.

Some medical schools around the United States did not include the teaching of normal and abnormal sleep in their cur-

Possible Signs of Sleep Problems

Check any of the following statements that describe you. Talk with your doctor if you check more than two.

- ☐ I have a headache in the morning upon getting out of bed.
- ☐ I feel scattered aches and pains throughout my body upon arising.
- ☐ I feel fatigue or tiredness that does not go away even after several large cups of strongly caffeinated coffee.
- ☐ I feel in a low mood that does not lift even as I get on with my daily activities.
- ☐ I have felt depressed enough to seek psychiatric help or to obtain antidepressant medications.
- ☐ I feel irritable, impatient, and moody.
- ☐ I often have an inability to maintain social harmony with family and friends.
- ☐ I have trouble learning new information or grasping new ideas.
- ☐ I am unable to recall useful information.

ricula until the 1980s. Therefore, many practicing physicians in the nation today have no knowledge or training in the areas of sleep disorders. In fact, the American Medical Association did not recognize sleep medicine as a specialty until 1996.

We knew very little about the behavior of sleep until the early 1900s, when researchers began to experiment with the light-dark cycle to show how it affected human behavior. These findings were followed with research in circadian behavior (the biological clock) and electrophysiology, which measured brain waves. Rapid eye movement (REM) sleep was first described in the early 1950s, and the first clinical sleep laboratories opened in the early 1970s.

What we do know is that there are distinct behavioral and physiologic changes in normal sleep with two specific sleep states: rapid eye movement (REM) and non-REM (NREM). Even though sleep is highly regulated by the body's homeostatic (internal equilibrium) and circadian processes, many factors affect its stages and duration; these factors include temperature, drug use, age, medical illness, and psychiatric disease.

Normal sleep is a restorative state of diminished arousal. When sleep is disrupted or inadequate, it can lead to increased tension, vigilance, and irritability. It is not unusual for someone whose sleep is disrupted to wind up in a vicious sleep-deprived cycle, resulting in irritability and fatigue during the daytime hours and tension and anxiety while tossing and turning at night.

Sometimes insomnia or difficulty maintaining sound sleep is a clear warning sign of a psychiatric disorder. As part of the National Institute of Mental Health Epidemiologic Catchment Area study, researchers interviewed a community sample of 7,954 individuals at baseline and 1 year later about sleep complaints and psychiatric symptoms. They found that individuals with insomnia at baseline were 34 times more likely to develop a psychiatric disorder (particularly unipolar major depression) in 1 year compared to individuals without insomnia. Forty percent of those patients with insomnia and 46.5 percent of those with hypersomnia already had a psychiatric disorder, compared with 16.4 percent of those with no sleep complaints. The researchers concluded that the risk of developing new major depression was even higher in those who had insomnia at both baseline and 1 year later than those without insomnia.[4] In addition, studies of patients who suffer with anxiety disorder and panic disorder have revealed a higher prevalence of sleep complaints than in patients without these psychiatric disorders.[5]

Because obtaining restful sleep is crucial for those with

Bipolar II disorder, it is helpful to understand the characteristics of normal sleep and how this differs from the sleep experienced by those who are bipolar.

CIRCADIAN RHYTHMS

Comprehensive scientific studies suggest that a complex system of nerve cells and interconnections within the brain are responsible for the cycles of sleep and wakefulness. We have a built-in cycle of sleep-wake times called circadian rhythms ("circa" means around, and "dia" means day). A group of nerve cells called the circadian pacemaker controls these cycles and is closely related to parts of the retina in the back of the eyes and the hypothalamus in the brain. The 24-hour cycle is an important organizing principle in our physiology, since body temperature, blood pressure, respiration, pulse, blood sugar, hemoglobin levels, and amino acid levels change according to this cycle. Strength and weakness also vary with the time of day. These fluctuations translate into a pattern of either early rising and morning alertness or staying up late and feeling most alert at night. We call the synchronized changes in internal body characteristics our circadian rhythms.

Circadian rhythms determine our daily sleep cycles, performance, alertness, moods, and even our gastrointestinal and metabolic functions. Scientific findings indicate that patients with bipolar disorder have less stable and more variable circadian activity patterns than do non-bipolar patients.[6]

The hormone most closely linked with the circadian system is melatonin, which is made by the pineal gland in the base of the brain. With sunlight, the body's primary timekeeper, melatonin helps to set the brain's biological clock. During the biological night, melatonin is secreted, the body temperature lowers, and sleep propensity increases.[7]

The circadian cycle is actually 25 hours long. Since this cycle is longer than the 24-hour day, some factors must serve to coordinate the body's pacemaker with the external clock. We adjust by using internal cues such as the body's biological clock, or the response to the amount of time since the last sleep episode, and external cues such as light or darkness, temperature changes, humidity and barometric pressure, and, perhaps, even eating patterns. Core body temperature has a 24-hour rhythm that supplies the internal timing for sleep and wakefulness. Sleep characteristically occurs when the temperature rhythm is declining, whereas wakefulness occurs when the temperature is rising.

The internal and external cues allow us to reset our circadian clock every day and adjust to changes that might throw us off, such as jet lag, sleeping in or staying up late, or working a night shift. These adjustments are not always easy, so symptoms can occur that indicate we are "out of sync," such as stomach upset, weakness, irritability, insomnia, or a shortened attention span. For those with Bipolar II, getting out of sync with their circadian clocks can precipitate hypomania, or even mania in some cases.

Under normal circumstances, we awaken in the morning in response to some cue such as an alarm clock (or in my case, three alarm clocks) or sunlight beaming through the bedroom window. As the morning hours advance, we get more alert until about 1:00 p.m. or 2:00 p.m., when we have a lull or sag in wakefulness. Although you may think this dip in alertness was caused by a large lunch, this is not so. The lull is a natural consequence of our circadian rhythm. Interestingly, some cultures, such as those in Latin America, Italy, parts of Southeast Asia, and the Middle East, incorporate this lull into each day's schedule by taking a siesta (or nap) in the early afternoon, then getting back to work later on. Later in the afternoon, we become more alert and energetic again until late evening, when we start to experience a wave of sleepiness. With our usual bedtime ritual, we fall asleep until the next morning, when the cycle starts again.

For years, scientists have wondered whether abnormalities in circadian rhythm regulation may be involved in mood disorders. Researchers have observed that sleep duration changes dramatically when bipolar patients cycle between depression and mania. Bipolar patients with depression also have hypersomnia, which is an inability to stay awake; sufferers sleep more than 10 hours on a regular basis for at least 2 weeks. When bipolar patients are manic, they experience total insomnia, or the inability to sleep. In a study from the United Kingdom, researchers at the University of Manchester found that bipolar patients had less stable and more variable circadian activity patterns than controls (persons without psychiatric illnesses). These circadian activity disruptions were apparent in the bipolar patient even when there were no symptoms at all.[8]

THE STAGES OF SLEEP

Invariably, sleep patterns are reliable indicators of whether a patient with Bipolar II disorder is likely to relapse or maintain remission in the near term. Regularly scheduled nightly sleep periods may be helpful in preventing rapid cycling in patients with hypomania, while the slightest irregularities in circadian rhythms may be warning signs of an approaching moodswing.

Distinct stages compose sleep, with each stage defined by brain waves, eye movements, and muscle tension. REM sleep takes place mostly during the last third of a night's sleep and normally composes 25 percent of the sleep period. During REM sleep, there are small, variable-speed brain waves and rapid eye movements like those of eye-open wakefulness, and there is no muscle tension. It is during REM sleep that we have most of our dreams. (When you are aroused from REM sleep, you may have recall of vivid imagery.) In NREM sleep, there are four different levels, or stages, characterized by different combinations of brain waves, eye movements, and reduced but not absent muscle tension.

- **Stage 1:** light sleep (transition from wakefulness to deeper sleep)
- **Stage 2:** intermediate sleep (40 to 50 percent of total sleep time)
- **Stages 3 and 4:** deep or slow wave sleep, also called delta sleep (10 to 20 percent of total sleep time)

The amount of delta sleep (stages 3 and 4) reflects a person's sleep quality, or intensity. This deepest level of sleep occurs mostly in the first third of the night and makes up about 10 to 20 percent of total nighttime sleep in normal young adults. Growth hormone secretion is highest during delta sleep, and some researchers believe that this stage is most important for growth and repair of body tissue.

As a rule, delta sleep decreases with age and may be brief in healthy, elderly males. With the process of aging, environmental noise throughout the nighttime hours usually arouses elderly adults because of their smaller proportions of delta sleep. Not surprisingly, young children have particularly large proportions of delta sleep, which increases if they become sleep deprived. This explains why waking up a young child can sometimes be difficult. Still, anyone who does not get enough delta sleep—no matter what age or gender—will feel tired and groggy the next day.

Accurate Diagnosis Leads to Proper Treatment

I have had numerous patients present with sleep problems who think they have a mood disorder, when all they really need is quality sleep. Then again, many people are misdiagnosed with a sleep disorder when, in fact, they have Bipolar II or major depression. For instance, the sleep rhythm in unipolar or bipolar depression often results in the patient feeling "low and slow" when they awaken. They are slow to process information; they're lethargic in movement; and any problem seems bleak. As they go through the day, however, they slowly improve. It is as if their bodies and minds begin to awaken as the day progresses, even if unexpected stressors hit. We refer to this as an a.m. diurnal rhythm. In contrast, in reactive depression, the patient usually feels great upon awakening. This early bird grabs the first worm, so to speak. As the day goes by, however, the reactive depressive person's mood state worsens as life knocks 'em down. We call this a p.m. diurnal rhythm.

Some researchers believe that neurochemical and neurobiological shifts cause the sleep disturbances associated with hypomania and depression. Still, we do not fully understand the biology that triggers sleep problems in those with bipolar disorder. In the following pages, I'll describe some common sleep problems associated with Bipolar II.

BIPOLAR DISORDER AND SLEEP

"How many hours do you sleep on average at night, and what is the quality of your sleep?" are two of the first questions I ask every patient on the initial interview and all subsequent follow-up visits. While the hypomanic usually gloats over how little sleep he needs, getting by on 3 to 4 hours a night, the lack of quality sleep can wreak havoc on his mood and decision-making abilities. Sleep deprivation results in feelings of malaise, poor concentration, and moodiness, and even accidental deaths.

In a revealing sleep study published in the September 2005 issue of the *Journal of the American Medical Association,* Judith Owens, MD, and her team of researchers from Hasbro Children's Hospital in Providence, Rhode Island, followed 34 pediatric residents from Brown University over the course of 2 years to compare post-call performance to performance after drinking alcohol. During this time, the residents were tested under light call (1 month of daytime duty with no overnight shift, or about 44 hours of work per week) and heavy call (overnight duty every fourth night with an average of 90 hours of work a week). The residents performed computer tasks to gauge their attention and judgment after their light call (after consuming alcohol) and heavy call shifts (with placebo). The residents who were on heavy call and had not ingested alcohol performed worse on the computer tests than those doctors who had taken alcohol and were on light call. Dr. Owens concluded that the residents were so sleep-deprived that they didn't recognize that their own judgment was impaired.[9]

Drugs, stressful situations, and even excessive noise can affect daily body rhythms and moods. Once a Bipolar II mood disorder with disturbed rhythms has begun, it tends to be self-perpetuating, since depression and anxiety are likely to disrupt 24-hour rhythms further. An irregular living schedule can aggravate mood disorders. The old-fashioned sanitarium rest cure was effective with the "nervous" because it put the patient on a regular schedule of sleep, activity, and meals.

Insomnia

How is your sleep? Do you have difficulty falling asleep? Or do you toss and turn most of the night until you fall into a deep sleep just hours before the alarm goes off? A person suffering from insomnia has difficulty initiating or maintaining normal sleep, which can result in non-restorative sleep and impairment of daytime functioning. Insomnia includes sleeping too little, difficulty falling asleep, awakening frequently during the night, or waking up early and being unable to get back to sleep. It is characteristic of many mental and physical disorders. Those with depression, for example, may experience overwhelming feelings of sadness, hopelessness, worthlessness, or guilt, all of which can interrupt sleep. Hypomanics, on the other hand, can be so aroused that getting quality sleep is virtually impossible without medication. In a study at the University of Oxford in the United Kingdom, Allison G. Harvey, PhD, and colleagues in the department of experimental psychology determined that even between acute episodes of bipolar disorder, sleep problems were still documented in 70 percent of those who were experiencing a normal (euthymic) mood at the time. These normal-mood patients with bipolar disorder expressed dysfunctional beliefs and behaviors regarding sleep that were similar to those suffering from insomnia, such as high levels of anxiety, fear about poor sleep, low daytime activity level, and a tendency to misperceive sleep. Dr. Harvey concluded that even when the bipolar patients were not in a depressive, hypomanic, or manic mood state, they still had difficulty maintaining good sleep.[10]

Delayed Sleep Phase Syndrome

This is the most common circadian-rhythm sleep disorder that results in insomnia and daytime sleepiness, or somnolence. A short circuit between a person's biological clock and the 24-hour day causes this sleep disorder. It is commonly found in those with mild or major depression. In addition, certain medications used to treat bipolar disorder may disrupt the sleep-wake cycle. I often recommend chronotherapy to patients. This therapy—an attempt to move bedtime and rising time later and later each day until both times reach the desired goal—is often used to adjust delayed sleep phase syndrome. To adjust the delayed sleep phase problem, sleep specialists might also use bright light therapy (see page 105) or the natural hormone melatonin, particularly in depressed patients.

REM Sleep Abnormalities

REM sleep abnormalities have been implicated by doctors in a variety of psychiatric disorders, including depression, post-traumatic stress disorder, some forms of schizophrenia, and other disorders in which psychosis occurs.[11] Special tests, called sleep electroencephalograms, record the electrical activity of the brain and the quality of sleep. From these tests, we know that in people who are depressed, NREM sleep is reduced and REM sleep is increased. Most antidepressant medications suppress REM sleep, leading some researchers to believe that REM sleep deprivation relates to an improvement in depressive symptoms.[12] Yet Wellbutrin XL, a common antidepressant, and some older medications used to treat depression do not suppress REM sleep. Researchers are therefore still trying to determine the connection between the REM sleep mechanism and depression.

Irregular Sleep-Wake Schedule

This sleep disorder is yet another problem that many with Bipolar II experience and in large part results from a lack of lifestyle scheduling. The reverse sleep-wake cycle is usually experienced by bipolar drug abusers and/or alcoholics who stay awake all night searching for similar addicts and engaging in drug-seeking behavior, which results in sleeping the next day. This sleep disruption and irregularity make it much more difficult for the bipolar patient's physician to treat him or her with conventional medications and adjunctive cognitive therapy. In most cases, the patient needs to acknowledge the drug-seeking behavior and get involved in a recovery program such as Alcoholics Anonymous, Cocaine Anonymous, or other group. Talk therapy with a psychologist is beneficial to many patients as they seek to change destructive lifestyle habits and learn new behaviors that will help them adhere to a more normal sleep-wake schedule.

SEASONAL PATTERNS

In 400 BC, Hippocrates gave some of the earliest recordings of seasonal rhythm disturbances when he stated, "Whoever wishes to investigate medicine properly should proceed thus: In the first place to consider the seasons of the year and what effect each of them produces."

Twenty-six-year-old Caitlin, an interior designer, came to my office one January, complaining of intense sadness and feelings of depression. She said that no matter how much sleep she got, it was never enough to knock out the pervasive fatigue, sluggishness, and low mood.

"Over the past few years, I have felt intense malaise for about 5 months of the year, during fall and winter," she told me. "I have no interest in my toddler or my husband, and I avoid answering the phone even when my twin sister or mother calls. I've turned down clients who have asked me to do freelance interior design work—something that I normally would love to do."

During the past winter months, Caitlin said that her appetite for carbohydrates greatly increased, and she gained almost 15 pounds. This made sense to me because carbohydrates boost serotonin, the soothing neurotransmitter in the brain, and the carbohydrates probably made her feel better briefly. She also noted that her ability to be productive decreased, as she spent mornings watching talk shows and afternoons staring at soap operas.

In trying to help Caitlin understand the possible reason for her moodswing, I explained the pathogenesis of seasonal affective disorder, or SAD. While not well understood, it is thought that the decreasing daylight available in fall and winter triggers a depressive episode in those people predisposed to develop this disorder.

Comforted to know she had a seemingly common disorder, Caitlin felt that this explanation was consistent with what she experienced each winter. She added, "When the arctic air takes a reprieve and springtime comes, I am myself again—outgoing, energetic, and completely interested in life. For the first time in months, I leave my apartment on Fifth Avenue and spend the day taking long walks with my child and friends. Then, in October, as the temperatures drop, I once again become a depressive recluse."

I explained to Caitlin that it is highly common for SAD to occur in both bipolar and unipolar disorders. Family and molecular genetic studies indicate that there may be a genetic link between seasonal variation in mood and SAD. We also believe that seasonal variations in mood and behavior are related to alcoholism, which often coexists with bipolar disorder (see page 119).[13, 14] While Caitlin did not appear to have bipolar disorder and had no apparent family history of mood disorders, I felt it was important for her to be aware of the link with SAD and alert me if she had further symptoms of depression or hypomania.

SAD can also occur in the summertime, as the story of Suki, the 38-year-old owner of a successful jazz club in New York City, illustrates.

Suki told me that she had a strong hypomanic state every spring followed by a major depression every summer. This is consistent with summer-onset SAD, which has been described in the medical literature as possibly being attributable to hormonal fluctuations, but the reasons are simply unknown at this time. Suki took medication to modulate her moods, particularly the summer depression. In fact, her moodswings became so predictable that she would mark her calendar a year in advance, as she had a tendency to go too "high" around the first week of April and too "low" the first week of June.

Three years ago, when seasonally triggered hypomania caused her mood to flare, Suki overextended her line of credit, neglected paying bills, and almost lost her business. It was at this time that she first came to see me for an evaluation and treatment. Since then, I've tried to educate Suki, during her infrequent visits, that she needs regular medication and year-round psychiatric monitoring to avoid moodswings altogether and to function optimally in business and in her personal life. But she continues to believe that she can manage her moodswings herself and promises to see me 2 weeks before she anticipates the high. The reality is that once the hypomania starts,

Suki actually craves the mild, unmedicated high. Only when she crashes into a deep depression in June, however, does she call me for professional advice and treatment.

Another patient, Lynda, a 35-year-old fashion merchandiser who was diagnosed with Bipolar II in her early twenties, is aware of the springtime link to her hypomania. As the days get longer, this former model finds that it is difficult to maintain normal sleep and feels revved up and hypersexual during this period. Lynda remembers being wound up so high a few years back that she had an impulsive one-night fling with an older man she met on a Caribbean cruise. She became pregnant and had to take a leave from her job because of medical complications associated with the pregnancy. While she adores her son more than life and the child's father (who had a family of his own at the time) pays generous child support, Lynda now has a better understanding of her Bipolar II condition and stays on mood-stabilizing medications year-round to help control her behavior and lifestyle habits.

It is thought that hormones, such as melatonin (see page 93), which are manufactured in the hypothalamus—the region of the brain that contains, among other things, the body's sleep, hunger, sex, and mood centers—may automatically trigger an attitudinal change at a certain time of year. We believe that hormonal changes are related to seasonal affective disorder; these biochemical fluctuations can also contribute to a summertime biological depression, similar to Suki's.

One of my former students at Columbia, Norman Rosenthal, MD, and his colleagues at the National Institute of Mental Health established the concept of SAD, characterized by recurring cycles of fall-winter depression and spring-summer hypomanias. Some cases of summer-onset SAD cause depression during the summer months and may be related to the higher temperature.

Those individuals with major depressive disorder or bipolar disorders often have comorbid seasonal affective disorder, as described in the *DSM-IV*. Studies indicate, however, that people with bipolar disorder experience greater seasonality of moods than those with recurrent depression, though the studies are too inconsistent to lead us to a definitive conclusion as to why. SAD causes seasonal highs and lows, and feelings of depression, fatigue, hypersomnolence, carbohydrate craving, weight gain, and loss of libido. Usually starting in young adulthood (around age 23), SAD is more common in women than in men and affects about 6 percent of Americans. An additional 10 to 20 percent may experience milder SAD symptoms. Because the lack of sufficient daylight during winter months may partially cause SAD, we seldom find it in countries within 30 degrees of the equator where the sun shines year-round. Many hypotheses exist regarding the biochemical mechanisms behind the predisposition toward this disease, including circadian phase shifting, abnormal pineal melatonin secretion, and abnormal serotonin synthesis.[15]

The exact pathogenesis of SAD is not well understood. I have Bipolar II patients who suffer depression every spring and fall, and most likely these low moods have a seasonal biological connection. The theory holds that a person's body chemistry determines spring moodswings—much like the menstrual cycle, which responds to certain hormonal clues in a clockwork fashion. Some mood-stabilizing medications and light therapy (see next page) for mildly depressed patients can help these moodswings.

If your depression appears to be seasonal in nature, regardless of what else is going on in your life, chances may be that you have a type of seasonal affective disorder. Moreover, as discussed on page 96, with most biological depressions, you may feel worse in the morning and better at night. Generally, environmentally or reactively caused depressions have the opposite effect. Antidepressant pharmacotherapy is often used as treatment for SAD, although researchers are continuing to find new therapies for resolving low mood.

DSM-IV Criteria for Seasonal Pattern Specifier[16]

A. "There has been a regular temporal relationship between the onset of major depressive episodes in Bipolar I or Bipolar II disorder or major depressive disorder, recurrent, and a particular time of the year (e.g., regular appearance of the major depressive episode in the fall or winter).

   Note: Do not include cases in which there is an obvious effect of seasonal related psychosocial stressors (e.g., regularly being unemployed every winter).

B. Full remissions (or a change from depression to mania or hypomania) also occur at a characteristic time of the year (e.g., depression disappears in the spring).

C. In the last 2 years, two major depressive episodes have occurred that demonstrate the temporal seasonal relationships defined in Criteria A and B, and no nonseasonal major depressive episodes have occurred during that same period.

D. Seasonal major depressive episodes (as described above) substantially outnumber the nonseasonal major depressive episodes that may have occurred over the individual's lifetime."

Light Therapy

Researchers have known for many years that when light strikes the human retina, the pineal gland is stimulated via neural pathways. This stimulation decreases the secretion of melatonin in the body. Some believe that it is highly possible that melatonin is related to depression in SAD patients and that light therapy has an antidepressant effect because it modifies the amount of melatonin in the nervous system. Other findings indicate that the neurotransmitter serotonin (see page 34) is involved in SAD and plays a role in therapeutic light therapy.[17]

An intriguing study from Finland researched the seasonal changes in mood and behavior and the persistence of the circadian rhythm in twins with bipolar disorder and their healthy co-twin (twin sibling). Researchers concluded that bipolar twins had greater seasonal changes in sleep length as compared with their co-twins with no psychiatric disorder. Interestingly, sunny days had a greater positive effect on well-being in the bipolar than the healthy co-twins, which supports the view that bipolar disorder is sensitive to environmental influences, in general, and to seasonal effects, specifically.[18]

Other scientific findings indicate that phototherapy (light therapy) may be effective treatment for bulimia nervosa, sleep maintenance insomnia, nonseasonal major depressive disorder, and some cases of bipolar depression. In one study, researchers gave only antidepressants to bipolar patients and noticed improvement of sleep and appetite, while bipolar patients who received antidepressants and light therapy reported the added benefit of increased energy and mood improvement.[19]

With light therapy, a person sits about 2 feet away from a very bright light, usually a 10,000-lux box, which is about 20 times brighter than normal room lighting. Patients initially use a 20- to 30-minute session per day. They increase this time gradually to 30 to 45 minutes a day, depending on the response. If symptoms are not resolved, the light therapy session increases to twice a day.[20] We believe that light therapy is effective in resolving between 60 to 90 percent of SAD cases. Those who respond to light therapy are encouraged to continue until they can be out in the springtime sun again.

The Amino Acid Tryptophan

For those patients who do not respond to light therapy for seasonal affective disorder, the amino acid tryptophan might hold some hope. Some revealing studies have been done on the therapeutic effects of light versus tryptophan on patients with SAD.

A. M. Ghadirian, MD, and his colleagues at Canada's McGill University assessed SAD patients at Royal Victoria Hospital who received light therapy for 2 weeks or tryptophan for 4 weeks. They found that while both therapies had a significant therapeutic effect, the relapse back into a depression occurred more slowly with tryptophan.[21]

In another study published in the journal *Psychology and Medicine,* A. Neumeister, MD, and colleagues at the University of Vienna in Austria established that SAD patients in remission during the summer months are more vulnerable to depression when their bodies are depleted of tryptophan. In this study, researchers gave SAD patients in remission two amino acid beverages—one containing tryptophan and the other containing no tryptophan. Dr. Neumeister found that patients who received the beverage with tryptophan had no alteration in brain serotonin and had no recurrence of symptoms. Yet those volunteers who received the tryptophan-free amino acid beverage had a transient return of depressive symptoms.[22]

It turns out that tryptophan is a precursor in the synthesis of serotonin in the brain—meaning, it's a biochemical substance that's necessary for the formation of the more stable serotonin. During the late 1960s and early 1970s, pharmacological studies suggested that the hormone serotonin might have a role in sleep induction. Later on, research in animals showed that destruction of the parts of the brain that housed serotonin-containing nerve cells could produce total insomnia. Partial damage to these areas of the brain caused variable decreases in sleep. The percentage of destruction of these particular nerve cells correlates with the amount of slow-wave sleep.

The influence of tryptophan on sleep continues to be studied in major sleep laboratories across the nation. While this amino acid is not available as a natural dietary supplement, it can easily be included in one's diet through foods such as turkey, cheese, nuts, beans, eggs, and milk, among others.

For Those with Bipolar II and Their Family Members

■ Because it is often difficult to initiate and/or maintain sleep with Bipolar II disorder, it is important to avoid stimulants such as caffeine and nicotine, especially near bedtime. Also check the ingredients in any over-the-counter or prescription medication to see if "sleeplessness" is indicated. Some seemingly innocuous medications such as headache remedies contain caffeine, which can result in poor sleep. Talk with your doctor if a change of medication is necessary.

■ Regular daily exercise, including stretching and aerobic activity, can help to consolidate sleep and alleviate the associated anxiety many have about staying asleep.

■ Because high levels of arousal associated with racing thoughts, worrying, or rumination may delay sleep onset, relaxation techniques such as yoga and deep abdominal breathing may be useful in initiating sleep.

■ Meditation, listening to soft music, or reading a book before bedtime may also help increase relaxation while focusing thoughts on a neutral or enjoyable target.

■ Avoid relying on prescription sleeping pills, if you can. Sleeping pills can sometimes lead to habituation or addiction—problems that may be more difficult to treat than the original problem causing the insomnia itself.

■ Although one night of disrupted sleep should not affect most Bipolar II patients, I have had patients who become hypomanic or manic after a single night of sleep deprivation. That is why it is important to keep lifestyle habits stable, sleep schedules regular, and medications at the optimal levels necessary to achieve mood stability and quality sleep.

CHAPTER 5

SEX, DRUGS, AND OTHER (MIS)BEHAVIORS

The much-publicized story of Mary Kay Letourneau and her grade school lover astonished millions. Married with four children, this young teacher found her calling in the public school classroom and took great pleasure working with exceptional or gifted children. One such student, Vili Fualaau, a student in her sixth-grade class, had an extraordinary artistic ability. Letourneau took Fualaau under her tutelage, and as the academic year advanced, so did their relationship, going from teacher-student to star-crossed lovers.

The two spent a lot of time together at Letourneau's home in the summer of 1996, and it wasn't long before Mary Kay was pregnant with Vili's child. In February 1997, after Fualaau admitted to authorities that he was having a sexual relationship with his teacher, Letourneau was arrested, handcuffed, escorted from the school, and charged with statutory rape. The scandal from the Seattle suburb hit the national news instantly, and people watched in sickened disbelief.

In March 1997, Letourneau pled not guilty, was released on bail, and was prohibited from seeing Fualaau, her 13-year-old lover. However, after she gave birth to their child, a girl, the young boy continued to visit his "teacher" regularly. In August 1997, Letourneau changed her plea to guilty of second-degree child rape and the case went to trial. A psychiatrist who took the stand gave more insight into Letourneau's behavior, saying that the woman had all the markers associated with the chemical imbalances in bipolar disorder, which can lead to irrational or irresponsible behavior. It was thought that Letourneau had severe hypomania during her relationship with the young boy.

The judge originally gave Letourneau a 7½-year prison sentence but reduced this to just 6 months, so she could seek treatment for her bipolar disorder. She was released from prison in January 1998 for "good behavior," but police caught Letourneau in a car with Fualaau just a month later. This time the judge did not grant leniency, the suspended sentence was revoked, and the original sentence was reinstated. Letourneau later discovered she was pregnant with the boy's second child (her sixth biological child). Her continuous defiance of the court's order to abstain from any contact with Fualaau led to 6 months in solitary confinement after the warden intercepted letters she had written to the young boy.

Today Letourneau is free and a registered sex offender. She and Fualaau are now married. In similar cases, two young female teachers—in Florida and Tennessee—were charged with having sex with their underage male students. In these cases, attorneys assert that the women have emotional illnesses that are not their fault.

I cannot overstate the importance of understanding the risky behaviors such as sexual indiscretions, substance abuse, and gambling that often co-occur with bipolar disorder. In this chapter, I will discuss these behaviors and elaborate on how they not only hurt the patient, but can cause significant distress for family members, friends, and co-workers.

Repeatedly, I have had urgent calls from distressed family members of bipolar patients pleading for help. Whether the misbehavior is sexual in nature, related to substance abuse, or because of an addiction to gambling or out-of-control credit card use, it is apparent that these high-risk behaviors frequently coexist in those who have Bipolar II disorder.

There are many theories on why some of these risky behaviors occur in bipolar illness. Most psychopharmacologists believe that the indiscretions represent a genetic connection. For example, an uncle had numerous sexual encounters, affairs, and failed marriages, and so the patient, who exhibits the same behaviors, is genetically like him. Or the grandfather and aunt were both alcoholics, so the patient's serious alcohol addiction must run in the family. Yet other experts contend that the risky behaviors are related to the patient trying to self-medicate his or her various moods, realizing that sex, alcohol, or recreational drugs, and even high-risk financial acts, can fan the fire of hypomania or numb the lows of depression. A few professionals consider the idea that risky behaviors coincide with the wide moodswings of bipolar disorder. For instance, a hypomanic person who feels highly energetic, positive, and elated may think nothing can go wrong if he or she gambles with the family's mortgage money—until the gambling deal turns sour. Or the depressed person with Bipolar II who masks his feelings with alcohol may not realize that, in reality, this is self-medicating a psychiatric illness—until that person loses his job or his spouse threatens to leave. No matter why these risky misbehaviors co-occur, they greatly complicate the diagnosis, treatment, and recovery for the patient with bipolar disorder.

For example, a 55-year-old woman named Jenny came to see me with her husband, David, who was in tears as he begged me to help his wife. From first appearance, Jenny seemed quite subdued and sophisticated. Still, I could not help but notice that this petite, shapely woman was sitting in a sexually revealing manner wearing a tight skirt and a low-cut blouse. With his wife by his side, David told me, "Over the past few weeks Jenny has been in what I call an off-the-wall hypersexual mood. She dyed her hair platinum blonde and had her ankle tattooed last weekend. Recently, at an office cocktail party, she was flirting with my male colleagues."

David described how Jenny "used to sleep 7 hours a night, but now is getting 4 to 5 hours of sleep. She has become extremely restless and is obsessively cleaning, exercising, or chatting with her sisters on the phone for hours each day."

Last week while he was watching television, David recalled that Jenny was scanning the Internet, looking at pornographic sites. "When I walked over to the computer, I noticed that she was talking to other men in a sex chat room. This sexual promiscuity is not like Jenny, who is normally very modest and cautious."

He added that Jenny had started demanding sex from him at least once or twice a day and even in the middle of the night while he was in a deep sleep. "When I cannot perform sexually or simply want to be left alone, she becomes outraged and even cries in anger," David said. "It's like she's on the sexual prowl, but this behavior is killing me—and our marriage."

Hypersexuality, as David described his wife's behavior, is common among those with Bipolar II disorder. I asked to speak with Jenny alone, and during our discussion, I noticed other behaviors that were consistent with Bipolar II's hypomania. For example, she was highly distracted, preferring to walk about my office examining and commenting on the artwork rather than sitting and facing me. She had slightly pressured speech, and her thoughts seemed to fly from one subject to another as she talked about their children, her new swimsuit, and a religious book she had just finished reading. "There is nothing wrong with me," Jenny said. "What's wrong with enjoying sex? The real problem is that David has just gotten old before his time."

From her symptoms of increased motor activity and energy, needing less sleep, flamboyant dressing, and hypersexuality, Jenny seemed to meet the established criteria for a Bipolar II mood disorder. In talking further about her medical history, she mentioned that she had once spoken to her primary care doctor about her moodswings and inability to sleep. Her doctor had asked Jenny if she had a history of depression or mood disorders but did not refer her to a psychiatrist. Instead, the doctor gave Jenny sleeping pills that made her feel overly drugged.

While patients who are manic often require hospitalization to stabilize their moods, individuals who are hypomanic such as Jenny can usually be treated on an outpatient basis with medications. Some require no treatment at all. With the support of David, I convinced Jenny that a small dose of a mood-stabilizing medication would help to calm the hypomania and allow her to feel more in control of her emotions, sleep habits, and life, in general.

A month later, Jenny came back for a follow-up visit and was in a noticeably calmer, more normal state of mind. The medication had moderated her excessive energy and hypersexual nature, and she was sleeping 7 to 8 hours at night. She felt rested, and her marital relationship was getting back to normal. Jenny reported no uncomfortable side effects from the medication and is still compliant with the treatment.

SEXUAL ADDICTION

Many adults feel flirtatious from time to time, particularly in social settings, but have enough self-control to know where to draw the line. Sexual compulsivity or addiction is different from being overly friendly at an office party. Defined as lack of control over one's sexual behavior, sexual compulsivity is becoming increasingly common among the general population and is often associated with considerable negative consequences. Sexual compulsivity appears in both men and women but may be more common in men. Patients with sexual compulsivity may be pathological in various behaviors, such as changing sex partners frequently, masturbating compulsively, and using pornography excessively. Years ago, we called a person who exhibited such addictive behavior a nymphomaniac or a Don Juan. Today we know the problem lies much deeper than the patient's outward hypersexual addiction.

With sexual addiction, you may feel highly flirtatious even with married co-workers or strangers you meet at the mall. As the person responds to you, you feel charged up, almost like you are "high." To illustrate this further, I will use the example of my patient Morgan, a young woman in her late twenties who lost her career and her marriage because of untreated Bipolar II disorder and out-of-control hypersexual behavior. The first time I consulted with Morgan, she told me, "My mother was diagnosed with bipolar disorder when I was 16, and my father was alcoholic, with moderate to severe depressions. I also had an aunt who had committed suicide in her thirties, and an uncle who had made millions as a stock trader. He was notorious in our family for his boundless energy as well as his heavy drinking."

Morgan said that she attended college in Pennsylvania, and by her senior year in college, she was president of the public relations club, was busy on student government committees, and chaired two sorority organizations that planned various fundraising activities, including group trips for spring break. "I met Richard, a senior engineering student at a nearby college, during spring break," she said. "We fell in love, and planned to get married after graduation. Up until that point, I had avoided the heavy drinking party scene. Then suddenly, I became fascinated with frat parties and was voted to be a 'little sister' for a popular fraternity on campus. Sometimes I had sex with a couple of guys from the fraternity all in a week."

Morgan said she felt on top of the world at that time, and her sexual habits were no different from many of her college friends, even though she drank more than her friends thought was good for her.

"After Richard and I got married, I started tutoring at a small religious school near our condo. In the first year of marriage, instead of being starry-eyed, I became very depressed and often had trouble getting out of bed in the morning. I gained about 20 pounds, and that added to my low mood. Richard didn't even notice how depressed I was as he was very involved in his graduate program."

After 2 years, Morgan said her depression appeared to lift and she became her talkative former self. She began to hatch grandiose plans for improving the house and the school where she worked, and she started three Internet sales businesses, which she worked on for several hours each evening. Richard was pleased that she seemed more interested in life, and she gathered a large circle of new friends with her talkative, open manner. Her Internet trading started to make good money.

During this initial consultation, Morgan told me about her recent sexual escapades, including her involvement with a man who had come to do repairs in the condominium where she and Richard lived. "We'd have sex several times in one afternoon," she said. "The more we had sex, the higher I felt, and the more I tested the limits. Besides having sex with him, I became sexually involved with one of the teachers at the school where I taught. Richard had no clue that this was going on, until he came home early one day and found the repairman there and became very suspicious."

Looking back, Morgan realized that she was living dangerously, in that she began having one-night stands with strangers or people she barely knew. She said that one of Richard's friends saw her with the teacher at a local club and told him what he had seen going on. "When Richard confronted me, I could not deny it, but I had to tell him up front that he was not enough for me. I felt this inner compulsion to have sex with many people, and I could not control it."

After listening to Morgan's lengthy bipolar history, I told her about Bipolar II with its depression and hypomania and how I felt that a long-term mood stabilizer would help balance her moodswings and maybe save her marriage and career. I also insisted upon adjunctive cognitive therapy and regular attendance at Sex Addicts Anonymous meetings. Morgan was surprisingly compliant and agreed to take the medication and get counseling.

As often happens, after 2 months of treatment, Morgan proclaimed herself well and discontinued the medication, counseling, and her involvement with Sex Addicts Anonymous. She began to feel better and quickly re-escalated into her hypomanic self. One night when Richard was out with colleagues, Morgan ran away, only to be picked up 300 miles away at a bus station. Richard took Morgan back to their apartment, and then he moved out the next day. By denying that she needed treatment for a serious mood disorder, Morgan risked losing her marriage, her teaching career, and her sense of self-worth.

Morgan is a tragic example of a bright young person with Bipolar II who, because of the illness not being diagnosed and treated soon enough, destroys her reputation, career, and marriage—and Morgan is not alone by any means. I've treated numerous patients with Bipolar I and II disorder who, during their risk-taking highs, are also driven higher by physical attraction, heightened sensory awareness, and their sexual addiction. Many of my patients with Bipolar II disorder say they feel sexier, more youthful, and attractive when their hypomanic mood escalates. When they switch into their highs, they do not have time to eat, so they quickly lose weight. This often leads to spending sprees to buy more sexy and flamboyant clothes to fit their smaller size and rediscovered hypersexual image.

When many hypomanics crave sex, most of the time it is not "safe" sex with their partners in a monogamous relationship. Many of my patients admit to having numerous sexual partners. Some suffer with unwanted pregnancies or sexually transmitted diseases, are addicted to online pornography sites, or stay up all hours into the night engaged in online chat rooms seeking sexual pleasure and partners. It is not unusual for those with Bipolar II to engage frequently in phone sex or sex with prostitutes who might have lethal health histories. I have patients with Bipolar II who are addicted to sex and have risked high-powered careers for a brief lunchtime fling with another colleague. Some have lost their life savings paying for that brief but pleasurable thrill. Perhaps the gravest situation is that many lose their marriages, careers, and the respect of their children and friends.

Perhaps the increase in sexual (mis)behavior is one of the least discussed indicators of a hypomanic state. Granted, an enjoyment of and appreciation for sexual relationships is quite normal and healthy. Pick up most books or magazines, turn on the television or radio, or log onto the Internet, and you will undoubtedly find sexual content. There certainly is an audience for this material, but when a normal enjoyment of sex becomes a Bipolar II hypersexual preoccupation or sexual addiction, it is time to seek professional help.

Most Bipolar II individuals who have hypersexuality to the point of an addiction do not recognize the ultimate dangers associated with this problem. I always ask my patients the following questions that are characteristic of sexual addiction to help them recognize the problem. Once we agree there is a problem, we discuss treatment protocols, including medications (see chapter 8). (If you answer yes to 5 or more of these 14 questions, you most likely have an addiction.)

1. Do you have obsessive thinking about sex all the time—more so than your friends?
2. How often do you have sex with multiple partners?
3. How often do you have sex with someone you just met that night?
4. How difficult is it to control your need to have sex irrespective of the person, the gender, or the consequences?
5. Do you have unsafe sex?
6. Do you feel little to no guilt for craving sex with partners outside of a monogamous relationship?
7. Has your spouse (or family members) left you because of your hypersexual addiction?

8. Have you ever had sex with a co-worker as an impulsive act?
9. Have you missed work because you were acting on your hypersexual need?
10. Have you conceived a child out of wedlock during a sexual escapade?
11. Have you contracted a sexually transmitted disease because of having unprotected sex?
12. Do you drink or use recreational drugs to make your sexual experience higher? How often?
13. Have you lost your job or income because of your sexual addiction?
14. Has your partner confronted you with the problem of sexual addiction?

The Hypomanic Prowl Leads to Sexual Addiction

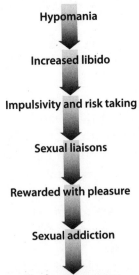

Hypomania

Increased libido

Impulsivity and risk taking

Sexual liaisons

Rewarded with pleasure

Sexual addiction

Final consequences
(including the breakup of marriages, unwanted
pregnancies, HIV/AIDS and other sexually transmitted diseases,
loss of job and income, depression, and sometimes legal suits and jail)

SUBSTANCE ABUSE

Not only do individuals with mood disorders have higher risks for episodic promiscuity, extramarital affairs, or a compulsion toward sexual encounters, they are also prone to alcohol or drug abuse as a way of self-treating the high anxiety during the down mood or augmenting the elation and energy during the hypomanic high. In fact, bipolar disorder is associated with the highest rate of substance abuse of any psychiatric illness, with almost two-thirds of men and women with Bipolar I and II meeting the diagnostic criteria for an addictive disorder. When people with bipolar disorder get depressed, they frequently try to drink or drug their undesired mood away, even if they are highly cognizant of their substance abuse problem.

The correlation between drugs and alcohol and psychiatric illness has been debated for centuries. Scientists believe that depression is associated with a decreased activity of important brain neurotransmitters such as dopamine and serotonin; the opposite is true for hypomania. As discussed on page 36, antidepressants increase the availability of these neurotransmitters in the brain's synapses, but so can illicit drugs.

In my practice, the comorbidity of Bipolar II and substance abuse is explosive, with alcohol the leading precipitator of depressive episodes in many of my patients who are genetically vulnerable for depression or bipolar disorder. In fact, approximately 15 percent of all adults who have a psychiatric illness in any given year also experience a co-occurring substance abuse disorder, which complicates treatment.[1]

Alcohol is a central nervous system depressant, which is why many people use it as a tranquilizer at the end of a hard day or as an assist for tense social situations. I have some patients who stop drinking when they are depressed, but it is more common that Bipolar II patients increase their alcohol intake during low moods. According to the National Institute of Mental Health Multisite Epidemiologic Catchment Area Study, people with bipolar disorder are five times more likely to develop alcohol misuse and dependence than the rest of the population. For women, Bipolar II is associated with a higher incidence of alcohol abuse than Bipolar I; the incidence is about equal for men.

Sometimes, in someone genetically predisposed to bipolar disorder, alcoholism will begin before Bipolar II symptoms appear. At other times, the person will harbor Bipolar II depression and hypomania, and prefer to use alcohol as a means of self-treatment. When a patient presents with both alcoholism and Bipolar II disorder, we use the term *dual-diagnosis*.

All psychoactive drugs have the potential of altering mood in those with Bipolar II. Cocaine and amphetamines are the leading substances that precipitate hypomanic episodes. Cocaine abuse is associated with a several-fold increase in the incidence of bipolar disorder; in fact, the rate of bipolar disorder in cocaine abusers may be higher than in any other category of substance abuse. Cocaine and amphetamines instantly flood the brain with dopamine, a key neurotransmitter that regulates mood, movement, attention, and learning. Some people with Bipolar II use hallucinogens and marijuana to reduce or suppress the symptoms of hypomania, while others self-medicate to enhance their hypomanic symptoms.

It is thought that the rate of overall substance abuse among those with Bipolar I and II disorder is as high as 60 percent; cocaine abuse is reportedly as high as 30 percent. Generally, men seem to have higher rates of comorbid alcohol abuse/dependence and cannabis abuse/dependence than women do. But Bipolar II patients who abuse alcohol or drugs usually have a worse outcome than Bipolar II patients who are not substance abusers. Similarly, those Bipolar II patients who have comorbid substance abuse problems are also 15 times more likely to commit suicide than those without dual-diagnosis.

A history of first-degree relatives is important in understanding a person's propensity for alcoholism and substance abuse. Relatives of alcoholics often likewise suffer from alcoholism, as well as suicidal behavior, serious depression, or moodswings. For example, there were many media reports about Rhode Island Congressman Patrick Kennedy, son of Senator Edward (Ted) Kennedy, undergoing treatment for cocaine abuse in 1984 when he was a student at Phillips Academy. Although Patrick disclosed in 2000 that he has sought treatment for mental illness, he became more specific in 2004 by openly disclosing that he suffers from bipolar or manic depression.

It would seem that alcoholism runs in the family. Patrick's brother, Edward Jr., has undergone alcohol treatment. Patrick and his siblings acknowledge that they have become legal guardians for their mother, Joan Kennedy, to help her receive continued treatment for her long-standing alcoholism. Joan was arrested three times for drunken driving in the 1980s and 1990s and has spoken publicly in the past about her disease and recovery. Of course, the media reports of Ted Kennedy's own alcohol problems have been ongoing for decades.

In the US House of Representatives, Patrick Kennedy has made mental illness one of his key issues, sponsoring legislation that seeks to compel insurance companies to cover mental illness as they would any other health problem.[2]

Other public figures have openly discussed overcoming a coexisting substance abuse problem with bipolar disorder. Actor and bodybuilder Jean-Claude Van Damme, who has manic depression, started doing cocaine in 1993. He admitted that at one time, he had an $8,000-a-week habit of 4 to 5 grams of cocaine a day, before checking himself into a rehab program in Marina del Rey, California. Today he uses medication to treat his bipolar disorder instead of abusing recreational drugs.[3] Actor and author Carrie Fisher is a staunch advocate and educator for bipolar disorder, with which she was diagnosed at age 24. Fisher contends that she did not accept this diagnosis until 4 years later, when an overdose of drugs almost killed her.[4] She endured a major breakdown in the late 1990s, thought to be precipitated from an allergic reaction to a medication. In retrospect, her mental breakdown is consistent with bipolar disorder and may have happened anyway if not properly treated. Today she has written several books, including *Postcards from the Edge* and *The Best Awful,* which give further insight into life with manic depression. Actor Linda Hamilton lived with untreated bipolar disorder for 20 years before she was diagnosed in 1995. At age 20, Linda turned to cocaine and alcohol to boost her confidence and keep her inner demons at bay. After failed marriages and years of depression, Linda now takes prescribed medication to stabilize her moodswings.[5]

As so many people have experienced, not only does substance abuse erode the personality, it increases the chance of broken relationships, failed marriages, job loss, and even suicide. In particular, cocaine produces acute panic and anxiety and can lead to a full-blown psychosis complete with hallucinations. Once a person becomes a chronic user, the only treatment that seems to work is Narcotics Anonymous (NA) or Alcoholics Anonymous (AA) and complete abstinence. Phasing out slowly, just cutting down, or substituting one drug for another (called cross-addiction) simply does not work.

For patients who use cocaine, I usually recommend an inpatient hospital program to increase their chances of succeeding in rebuilding a drug-free life. This program requires time in a treatment center, with group and individual counseling, peer group meetings, and Cocaine Anonymous meetings, along with NA and AA.

For individuals who are addicted to alcohol, I recommend AA, which has been proven the most effective method worldwide to treat severe alcoholism. When I first begin treating bipolar patients with alcoholism, in addition to prescribing mood-stabilizing medication, I insist that they go to AA on a daily basis in the beginning. They also must choose a mentor outside of AA whom they trust and then meet with that person daily for the first few weeks or, in some cases, much longer. While the medications and the adjunctive psychotherapy take over, I insist on meeting the spouse or any other first-degree relative to strengthen the overall educational-support system. If the person is too sick from depression, mania, or an attempted suicide in combination with the alcoholism, then the patient should be hospitalized in a dual-diagnosis ward where treatment and withdrawal can be managed alongside the bipolar medications.

To identify potential problems with substance abuse, I discuss questions similar to the following with my Bipolar II patients. (If you answer "yes" to 5 or more of these 19 questions, you most likely have a problem with substance abuse.)

1. Do you use alcohol or recreational drugs daily?
2. Do you ever drink or use drugs during the morning hours?
3. Do you drink or use drugs while at work?
4. Do you miss work because of drinking or using drugs? How often?
5. Do you have problems controlling your urge to drink or use recreational drugs?
6. Do you use income intended to pay household bills to purchase alcohol or drugs?
7. Have you missed paying your mortgage because of your need to buy alcohol or drugs?
8. Have you lost your home because of this addiction?
9. Have you lost your job because of this addiction?
10. Has your spouse left you because of drinking or using drugs?
11. Do you turn to alcohol or drugs when you are feeling depressed or let down?
12. Do your friends know that you use alcohol or drugs or are you secretive?
13. Has this addiction shattered relationships with family members and friends?
14. Has the drinking or drug addiction injured your physical health?
15. Have you ever had an accident (automobile or other) because of the substance abuse?

16. Do you experience blackouts because of substance abuse?
17. Have you had times where you don't remember how you arrived home the next morning?
18. Do you use alcohol to come down off a stimulant high (cocaine)?
19. Do you find yourself using drugs more frequently during periods of high and low moodswings?

BUYING SPREES AND GAMBLING

Along with sexual indiscretions and comorbid alcohol and substance abuse, many with Bipolar II seek help only after they have recklessly spent their life savings or made wild bets on the stock market—and lost. It is not unusual for hypomanics to go on wild shopping sprees, spending money they do not have (by running up debt on credit cards) and buying items they never intend to use but want more than anything at the time of the purchase. For instance, I will never forget the patient who came to our first appointment carrying a duffel bag filled with more than 100 pairs of white tennis socks!

I asked Veronica, a 31-year-old retail fashion buyer with Bipolar II, to write down her thoughts and feelings when she was unable to restrain herself from overspending. She wrote the following:

"When I start feeling that hypomanic 'buzz,' I never worry about earning money. Instead, I become intent on spending as much as I want. It is not unusual for me to run up my credit card debt in excess of 15 to 20 thousand dollars over a period of 2 or 3 weeks during this mental state. I buy anything and everything I see without regard to whether I need it or will use it. For example, last spring when I was experiencing a mild high, I booked a 2-week Mediterranean cruise for myself and two girlfriends. I didn't even ask my friends if they could get off work at that time. I then realized that I had nothing to wear on the cruise and charged about $6,000 in resort wear, including two evening gowns for the late-night formal dinners. Looking back, I see how extravagant and emotionally based the spending was, especially when I found out my friends could not go and my credit cards were over their limits. But at the time, it seemed the right thing to do—get what I wanted to soothe my hypomanic state, and try to impress my friends at the same time."

Compulsive spending is regarded as a problem with impulse control. At times, the hypomanic individual may be right on the brink of being out of touch with reality. An extreme example of this is a patient of mine who threw $50,000 out of his office window in midtown Manhattan and then called his bank to send over more money. Of course, the bank did not comply with his request, and my patient was later treated with a mood stabilizer to modulate his hypomanic mood state. Sure, this is a rare example, but it really did happen. And is there really any difference between tossing thousands of dollars "to the wind" and the compulsive gambler who loses all of his money in risky investments? Sadly, either might in consequence try to commit suicide—and succeed.

We believe that many hypomanics have the same components as what some psychologists label a "Type-T," or thrill-seeking personality. This personality dimension refers to individual differences in stimulation seeking, excitement seeking, thrill seeking, arousal seeking, and risk taking.[6] Whether he or she chooses the stock market, the racetrack, a poker game, or an all-nighter doing slots in Las Vegas, the hypomanic seeks excitement, craves the adrenaline rush, and thrives on the tension. When he loses, he starts again with a bigger and better plan to win. He finds that this form of instant gratification suits his hyperalert, fast-moving, impulsive temperament. And why not? I mean, with a real job, you have to clock in daily and wait 2 weeks for a bona fide paycheck. With high stakes at the racetrack, your winnings are instantaneous—or far too often simply nonexistent.

As I explained in *Moodswing,* when hypomanics are making a fast deal, they feel in control. They love the sensation of power and the thrill of winning. Usually, the money is secondary—something to have in case you need to eat. The real high comes from the thrill of the gambling itself—and most try to beat the system until their last day. But while gambling is a high for the hypomanic, it can lead to far-reaching consequences at work and in the family.

The problem of gambling with Bipolar II has escalated greatly with unlimited access to gambling facilities and day-trading accounts on the Internet. When the hypomania goes too high, the compulsive gambler may look for new ways to win money.

But why should someone get so depressed over money, one might ask; many people have repeatedly made and lost fortunes. But the psychiatrist wonders which came first in a financial disaster: Was it the chemical moodswing to a deep depression, or was it the actual loss of the fortune that prompted such a severe reaction? I maintain that the hypomanic high often prompts a reckless loss of money, and suicide is a consequence of what is now called double depression: the combination of the depression, which would have occurred once the mania subsided, and the depressive reaction to loss.

Many people do not realize that they have a gambling problem until they lose everything. That's why an open discussion with a psychiatrist or other professional may help the person own up to the problem and seek intervention. When Bipolar II patients come to my office presenting with a possible gambling problem, I ask them the following questions. (If you answer "yes" to 5 or more of these 16 questions, you most likely have an addiction.)

1. Do you gamble for money frequently?
2. Do you regularly bet on sports games?
3. Have you ever used a bookie?
4. Do you regularly use slot machines or other "devices"?

5. Do you bet on the lottery frequently?
6. Did anyone in your immediate family have a problem with gambling?
7. Do you feel guilty for gambling?
8. Have you borrowed money to gamble?
9. Have you neglected paying your mortgage or food bills to gamble?
10. Have you missed work because of gambling?
11. Have you ever overextended, gambling more money than you actually had?
12. Has gambling ever led you to consume alcohol or recreational drugs?
13. Do you receive criticism from a spouse or friend for gambling?
14. Have you stolen money to gamble?
15. Have you prostituted yourself to get money for gambling?
16. Have you had to borrow money to pay back gambling debts?

Treatment goals for Bipolar II patients who are pathologic gamblers are consistent with treatment for major affective disorders, alcoholism, or substance abuse, in that the psychiatrist works on restoring to the patient a normal way of thinking and living. Behavioral therapy is used to improve the patient's social skills, and cognitive-behavioral therapy may help the patient prevent relapse. Intervention to reduce the risk of suicide is also necessary.

COMORBID BEHAVIORS COMPLICATE DIAGNOSIS AND TREATMENT

For the hypomanic Bipolar II patient, there are three urgent needs that often trigger comorbid behaviors or even addictions.

1. **The need for immediate gratification.** The behavior (whether sex, abusing alcohol or drugs, or gambling) offers immediate gratification. It is a short-term, self-perceived benefit (the "high") for a higher long-term risk.

2. **The need to act impulsively.** Impulsivity, or the failure to resist an internal drive or stimulus, drives many Bipolar II patients into risky behaviors—and many often regret the action after it is over. In my experience, this is a core behavior in many patients with bipolar disorder.
3. **The need to take the high even higher.** When a person is hypomanic and wants to go even "higher," he may turn to stimulants, painkillers such as Oxycontin (oxycodone HCL) or Vicodin (hydrocodone-acetaminophen), cocaine, diet pills, or caffeine. When the hypomanic high becomes dysphoric (mixed with anxiety and physical exhaustion from no sleep), the person often self-medicates with alcohol or marijuana to come down.

Along with hypersexuality, substance abuse, and financial indiscretions, some people with Bipolar II disorder also exhibit compulsive kleptomania, which is the recurrent failure to resist the need or impulse to steal items even when they may not be needed for personal use. Kleptomania is an impulsive act that fulfills the person's need for immediate gratification. Many individuals with kleptomania get a pleasurable "high" from stealing, which pushes their mood even higher.

Elizabeth Anne, a 40-year-old heiress with Bipolar II disorder, has been repeatedly caught stealing from some of New York City's high-end clothing stores. As Elizabeth Anne explained to me, "I could buy the entire store, if I wanted. But hiding an article of clothing or a purse in my coat or bag and then trying to get through the door without getting caught gives me an incredible adrenaline rush. When I succeed, I'm on a 'high' for days. When I'm caught, I always vow never to do this again, until I'm feeling invincible again."

As Elizabeth Anne experienced, the excitement of kleptomania and the feeling that "I got away with this" fans the Bipolar II hypomanic mood and pushes it even higher.

There are also those Bipolar II individuals who are compulsive about traveling and must be on the go constantly. Whether speeding up the body with drugs, sex, travel, fast cars, compulsive stealing, or even highly emotional talking like some televangelists, the urgent needs of having immediate gratification, acting on impulsivity, and taking the mood even higher with risky behavior are consistent with many who have Bipolar II disorder. I will always wonder if charismatic televangelist Jim Bakker was in a hypomanic state when he lavishly spent millions of dollars of viewers' contributions to his ministry on himself and his family before being indicted for fraud and ending up in prison.

For Those with Bipolar II and Their Family Members

- Individuals with mood disorders often have a propensity towards some risky behaviors, including hypersexuality, substance abuse, gambling, and buying sprees. Being aware of this propensity can alert you and your family members to intervene and stop the behavior and then seek professional help before someone is hurt or money is lost.
- No matter what the coexisting behavior or addiction, it is vital that the person with Bipolar II admit to the addiction or problem and seek ongoing professional help with a psychopharmacologist or psychiatrist.
- Joining a support group is part of the treatment for addiction. You can search for specific support groups such as Alcoholics Anonymous, Cocaine Anonymous, Gamblers Anonymous, and Spenders Anonymous, and fellowship support groups such as Sexaholics Anonymous, Sex Addicts Anonymous, Sexual Compulsives Anonymous, and Sex and Love Addicts Anonymous. The only requirement for membership in any of these face-to-face support groups is a desire to stop the addictive behavior and get well.
- Along with the support group, continue to see your doctor regularly, engage in psychotherapy, if needed, and stay on your medications. Even the most compulsive, addicted person with Bipolar II disorder can turn his or her life around and gain control of the initial bipolar problem—if he or she stays committed to the plan of action for recovery.

CHAPTER 6

THE HYPOMANIC ADVANTAGE OF BIPOLAR II BENEFICIAL

While depression is the most common psychiatric or emotional problem for which people seek help, I believe that most doctors have failed to recognize the benefits of the softer form of bipolarity. Hypomania can be a heightened, ebullient mood characterized by indefatigable physical energy, a flood of ideas, and—more often than is usually credited—profound accomplishment.[1] It is the positive energizer that drives some of the most exuberant, creative, and productive overachievers in the world.

Without exception, every diagnosis in the *DSM-IV* implies a disorder, a deficit, a malfunction, or a problem of some sort. In previous chapters, I have described some of the serious problems that often coexist with Bipolar II disorder, such as sleep deprivation, hypersexual behaviors, gambling, and the high incidence of comorbid alcohol and substance abuse. Yet after treating hundreds of extremely successful people with bipolar disorder, I know there is a positive side to Bipolar II and developed the concept of Bipolar IIB ("B" stands for "beneficial"). I published the first scientific paper in 1992 on this subtle subtype of manic depression in which someone uses the hypomanic mood to great advantage, and I believe that one day Bipolar IIB will be included in the *DSM-V* or *DSM-VI* alongside Bipolar I and II.

Of course, the downside of Bipolar IIB is the presence of periodic depression, as I've previously discussed, which is often detrimental to self and others. But with the right awareness and treatment of periodic depression, I have seen in my psychiatric practice that Bipolar IIB can produce the best of what human beings can contribute to society. And while not all individuals with Bipolar II are geniuses, I'd estimate that without some form of Bipolar II hypomania, there would be fewer geniuses! When you combine ability and higher education with hypomania, you often have the combination for tremendous accomplishment and great achievement.

Still, we usually tend to stereotype those with psychiatric disorders and view them in a negative way. It is my hope that with re-education, we can come to appreciate the tremendous gifts that many people with this beneficial subtype of Bipolar II disorder have to offer, and that these people can learn to use the traits to their utmost advantage.

UNDERSTANDING THE BIPOLAR IIB ADVANTAGE

Over the past several decades, I would estimate that as many as a third of my patients with Bipolar II have been some of the most talented and able men and women in New York City. Unlike Bipolar I mania where a person's thoughts become jumbled and progressively worsen as the episode develops, my Bipolar IIB hypomanic patients tell of thinking with ultimate clarity and harboring feelings of exuberance, confidence, and enthusiasm. Instead of allowing the inexhaustible mood state filled with energy and ideas to hinder their productivity, they use it to their full advantage. A typical example of this comes from 37-year-old Jake, a Bipolar IIB patient of mine who owns a successful high-end furniture chain in the Northeast. Jake wrote this account a few years ago:

"About twice a year, I wake up long before the alarm goes

off and immediately know that my hypomania is back. Something about this elevated mood and accelerated thinking excites me. With hypomania, I think clearer. My mind is a wellspring of creative ideas—how to increase sales, how to motivate my sales team, and ways to market my furniture more effectively. Unlike racing, jumbled thoughts, these ideas are organized but unending. When I catch the train to Manhattan, I capture these ideas, writing them down, page after page, and then prioritizing them. I usually call an early sales meeting upon arrival at the office, and I start discussing my ideas with my employees, delegating tasks when I can, so we can act on these quickly. Invariably, a few weeks later, I look back and realize that the very ideas developed in my hypomanic state are the ones that motivated my staff to work harder, gave us the momentum to bring in new clients and contracts, and brought in tens of thousands of dollars in sales revenue. For me, being Bipolar IIB is a godsend. Sure, I have my share of depressed episodes. Somehow, I manage to 'ride' them out with a few lifestyle changes and medications. I long for the beneficial hypomania, which for years has fueled my most productive and creative undertakings."

Up to this point, I have discussed many of the serious problems associated with Bipolar II disorder, including the risky behaviors that often destroy relationships and result in loss of job or income. I now want to elaborate on the positive side of Bipolar II, what I call Bipolar IIB (beneficial). After reading this chapter, you will be enlightened in how those with Bipolar IIB are truly the "movers and shakers" of society. An understanding of the positive side of Bipolar IIB disorder can help you or your loved one feel confident in using these attributes to benefit yourself, your family, and society.

BIPOLAR IIB HALLMARKS

With insight and treatment, if necessary, those with Bipolar IIB can use the mild mania to attain great accomplishments. Let's look at some specific hallmarks of Bipolar IIB, which include being bold and adventuresome, successful and driven, gifted and entrepreneurial, exuberant and confident, highly productive with an antipathy towards sleep, controlling but cool, chatty and persuasive, intuitive and captivating, and charming and creative.

Bold and Adventuresome

Upon completing Harvard Medical School, I debated whether I would live in Boston, the educational capital of the United States, or go to New York City, the business, law, and artistic capital. I gave in to the desire to go to the Big Apple. New York attracted me because it represented tremendous numbers of cultures and stimuli. I was fascinated by the fact that the sidewalks were not wrapped up at 9:00 p.m. and life continued on all night, 24 hours a day, 7 days a week.

As I was mulling over the decision of where to pursue my psychiatric resident training and later set up practice, I picked up an essay by Pulitzer Prize–winning author E.B. White, who cowrote *The Elements of Style* and who at the time worked for Harold Ross at *The New Yorker.* In the essay, entitled "Here Is New York," White wrote of three types of New Yorkers: the man or woman who was born in New York, the New York commuter from surrounding cities, and the person who was born somewhere else but who came to the Big Apple in search of the arts, entertainment, and its exuberant immigrant spirit. After reading White's essay, my mind was made up: New York was clearly where I wanted to pursue the next phase of my education and life.

Now, after residing in New York for 3 decades, I can attest to the fact that New York is a conglomerate of hypomanic Bipolar IIB people who are often restless in their small towns and, therefore, ultimately leave for New York to indulge in limitless possibilities and experiences.

By their very nature, those with Bipolar IIB were the immigrants of the 1800s, the triumphant dreamers and inventors who have the ability to take great risks. They are the optimists, the idealists, the ones whose innovation brings them success in life. Whereas most people avoid taking risks or launching out with an unproven idea or theory, those with Bipolar IIB usually throw caution to the wind and confidently go with the unknown, somehow making it work in their favor.

An interesting theory by John D. Gartner, PhD, is that the United States is notoriously hypomanic *because* it is populated by immigrants, those very people who had the optimism, will, and adventuresome spirit and energy to leave their homes abroad and take the giant leap into the unknown. Think about it! If you are highly curious, energetic, and a risk-taker, you are more likely to tackle the unknown[2] than someone with low energy who rarely takes risks.

Bipolar IIB hypomanics are thrill-seeking, daring, and thrive on conquering the unknown. Perhaps the pioneers who led the wagon trains across America to settle in uncharted territories were characteristically hypomanic in nature. Today's astronauts are living examples of that immigrant spirit. These brilliant scientists are bold and self-confident, and they must crave risk. Although this is just an assumption, as a psychiatrist, I have to ask myself, who would want to fly to the moon unless he or she is at least a little hypomanic? Yet who can deny that these brilliant space explorers use their hypomanic adventuresome spirit to its fullest advantage to benefit the whole of society?

Successful and Driven

When I first started my psychiatric practice, I treated a number of prominent New Yorkers for ordinary recurrent depression. I remember one patient, Marian, a 39-year-old investor who had made millions in the futures market. While she sometimes experienced periods of depression, after an effective course of anti-depressants, this highly intelligent woman would suddenly snap back to what I considered to be "normal" mood. At that time, little was known about Bipolar II or hypomania. So, I would write the following note on her chart: "Marian is now well and stabilized from her depression." I did not realize at the time that Marian's "well" periods were really mild highs or productive and enjoyable. What I did witness repeatedly was that this incredibly gifted woman soared during her "well" periods, quickly moving to the top in her field and making a repeat fortune in the stock market for herself and others. Today, I would write on her chart the diagnosis of Bipolar IIB.

It is quite common for a person on a hypomanic high to think they feel great because the depression is finally over. Yet I've seen these feelings of elation (and relief) often push patients too high, and it is only when they use poor judgment with money or sex, or make a deal that totally collapses, that I realize the elated mood was more than sheer happiness. That's when it becomes obvious that I was dealing with a clear-cut case of the milder form of manic depression. After observing the "well" states of hundreds of patients with Bipolar II, I began to wonder what was so bad about being a mild manic-depressive if one could feel so exuberant and achieve so much. These mild to moderately high hypomanias allowed many of my patients to become superhustlers between their depressions, and in a society of hustlers, which New York City is, these men and women usually rose to the top.

Most hypomanics do not like anything or anyone to be slow, from their cabdrivers to their administrative assistants to the waiters at their favorite restaurants. They are genetically wired to move fast, think fast, and talk fast, and in so doing, they sometimes irritate those around them. Hypomanics want results—and they want them now. Many move up the chain of command by being charming, upbeat, talkative, seductive, and energetic. Others gravitate toward the top of organizations, even when lack of tact with colleagues might sabotage their advancement.

Sometimes those with Bipolar IIB are so literally driven that they tend to be highly aggressive and even hostile in their driving habits. Road rage is a prime example of a hypomanic taking his aggressive behavior too far. These violent acts can include impulsively ramming another car to "get even," intentionally switching lanes to trap another motorist, or even physically confronting another motorist in a fit of anger. Somehow, these irritable and angry individuals allow their moodswings to get in the way of common sense and the law.

Nadia is highly successful and appears to be driven in every area of her life. Right out of college, she was accepted into a high-powered MBA program, where she became a star and a favorite of her professors because she is extremely bright and intense. She showed a passion for study, was great at organizing among her classmates, and showed a real talent for innovative thinking and planning. When she and fellow students spent a month in Belize to enjoy the nightlife, Nadia brought her laptop along and reviewed material for the upcoming semester. When she graduated from the MBA program, she landed a great job at a well-known dot-com giant. Nadia is now 33. In spite of her company's male-dominated management, she has done extremely well and is in senior management today.

Even people who think Nadia is too aggressive have to admire her stamina. She has the ability to work an 80-hour week and to stick with getting a project approved even against board opposition. She admits to getting irritable easily, although fear of consequences usually keeps her in check. She is known to be somewhat hard on her secretaries and research assistants, because she doesn't know the meaning of "slow down." Because Nadia is so hypomanic, some of her colleagues think she has a form of attention deficit disorder, which she does not.

In fact, Nadia is a classic example of a Bipolar IIB, because she has the biochemical advantage of being in a mild high much of the time. That's not to say she hasn't seen the downside of manic depression. Twice in her life she's suffered from moderate depressions. They weren't bad enough to require hospitalization, but during her first depression, she did see her internist, who gave her one of the newer antidepressants at the time. She came to see me during her second depression, when she reported that she felt exhausted, anxious, unable to sleep or eat, and worst of all, in her mind, unable to keep up her hectic schedule because of chronic fatigue and low mood. When I suggested she might have a mild bipolar cycle, she explained that she thought both of her depressions actually were the result of overwork and exhaustion.

Like so many with Bipolar IIB, Nadia is very perceptive and intuitive about other people. At work, her perceptiveness about colleagues is legendary. But also like many with Bipolar IIB, she doesn't seem to have much understanding of herself. In fact, to some of her co-workers, she seems to be emotionally underdeveloped and a classic workaholic. Most of her intimate relationships suffer because of her inability to let down her guard, and her love life is a continuing saga of liaisons with powerful men. She just does not seem to have enough time when she's not working to establish a long-term relationship. Nonetheless, men are drawn to her incredible energy, and she does think that she'd like to settle down and start a family someday. But with her overly committed career, she would need one if not two au pairs in order to have children and still keep up with her frenetic schedule! Her frequent-flier miles are through the roof, with the business trips (almost every week), the vacation home she is having built in Belize, and the jaunts to Europe with one man or another.

Nadia is exceptionally charismatic and, consistent with Bipolar IIB, has that special gleam in her eyes that signifies curiosity and energy. If you met her, you'd think she was incredibly seductive and charming and very driven to succeed. If you followed her daily schedule, you'd see that she sleeps only about

3 or 4 hours a night, and you'd note that she doesn't seem to miss the sleep. She has a clear-cut advantage over her colleagues, who don't have all this time to follow up on minute details. Her biochemical advantage has made it possible for her to succeed in a big way.

Nadia's family history is also typical for a successful Bipolar IIB. Her parents divorced when she was young. Her father, an alcoholic, lives on caffeine and cigarettes to get a daily buzz. Her mother is a chronic gambler who enjoys frequent trips to Las Vegas. There is depression in the family, as well. Her older brother has been hospitalized for depression twice, though he does not have highs, as far as anyone has noted. While some friends believe that Nadia's drive is a form of compensating for her broken home, it is in fact the result of her biochemical advantage. Nadia is likely to continue to do well, with the chance that a moderate depression may recur, possibly every few years.

Personnel offices often seek out this Bipolar IIB individual— the kind of person who has an upbeat approach to things, who is a workaholic, an overachiever, overactive, and overproductive, and who is full of creative ideas. And if they don't go crazy over the top or retreat into the pits of depression, so long as their judgment is not impaired or they are surrounded by people who can keep them from going over the edge with disastrous business decisions, these are often the ideal people with which to staff a very productive office. They are envied by their colleagues unless their hypomania goes too high and they make poor decisions or a depression washes over them. Then they accomplish nothing . . . or they get into trouble with bouts of anger, sexual harassment, or fraudulent business deals.

Gifted and Entrepreneurial

While I attest that making an "armchair" psychiatric diagnosis is subject to error and usually suspect, nonetheless, I fully believe that individuals with Bipolar IIB are in the media virtually every day—some diagnosed, many not. You hate to label people, but the roller-coaster existences of many tycoons whom we read about in the *New York Times* and in *Forbes* and *Fortune* magazines are not dissimilar to what you'd see in my patients who have Bipolar IIB. These extremely successful entrepreneurs are motivated by their hypomanic energy and exuberance.

The entrepreneur with Bipolar IIB is characterized by working long, hectic days with little sleep, nonstop talk, risky deals, and boundless energy—traits that mark some of our nation's highest-profile business leaders—abruptly truncated by plunges into bleak depression. I've treated numerous highly successful hypomanic entrepreneurs in New York who claim they never get depressed. I originally described the hypomanic entrepreneurs in 1975 in my book, *Moodswing,* as having the Midas touch.[3] Most of these fast movers see depression as a character weakness or a stigma that may injure their reputation among colleagues. Sometimes, only their spouses or their colleagues at the office who know them well see this downside, and it never gets reported. Perhaps you can think of a publicly elected official who suddenly takes a month off for personal reasons. Or what about the popular university professor or famous TV evangelist who quietly takes a sabbatical for "rest"—or jail? Many times these vibrant hypomanics have come down from their highs and fallen to their lowest point. Rather than being open about their illness, they sneak away for attempts at self-stabilization.

Hal was one of my friends from my time at Harvard Medical School. After graduating from Harvard Law, he bypassed paying his dues with the usual 80-hour work weeks for 15 years in a Wall Street firm and went straight to Venezuela to make a fast fortune in the timber business. To say Hal was driven was putting it mildly. After he made a lifetime fortune in less than 5 years, I would see Hal from time to time in New York restaurants and at private parties. He was always the "star"—the fast-talking center of attention, the one who could make action happen just by being in the room. After a few years, I heard that Hal was working overseas, buying and selling property.

Hal knew of my research in lithium and manic depression at Columbia. Yet I heard little from this man until I got a most curious phone call in the middle of the night from Japan.

"Ronnie, this is Hal. Say, Ronnie, how much lithium does a manic-depressive have to take to control his highs and lows?" I told Hal that the average is about 900 to 1,200 milligrams a day. He said a brief "thanks" and quickly hung up the phone without so much as a good-bye or any explanation for the call.

I didn't hear from Hal again until 4 years later. Again, it was the middle of the night, and this time I got the call from Moscow. "Ronnie, it's Hal. I have a question. When you take lithium, what's the therapeutic blood level you want to achieve?" I answered that it should be around 0.5 to 1 milliequivalent per liter. Again, he said, "Thanks, Ronnie," and hung up the phone without any further conversation.

Last year, Hal was back in New York with wife number four, and he invited me and my wife to his private Fifth Avenue club for lunch. As I was sitting next to him in his stretch limousine, listening to his ostentatious stories of how he had made millions in Moscow oil deals, I could not help myself from interrupting him and asking what had been on my mind for years: "By the way, Hal, do you ever get depressed?" His response was revealing. "Oh, no, Ronnie, never depressed, but sometimes I do lose my enthusiasm."

For a hypomanic who thrives on being driven, "losing their enthusiasm" is, in my mind, definitely equivalent to a minimal to mild depression!

CNN founder and philanthropist Ted Turner, often tagged the "flamboyant billionaire," has openly acknowledged that he has bipolar disorder. Through his vision, Turner changed the face of global awareness and created a multibillion-dollar empire in communications after first winning America's Cup. When Turner founded CNN, today one of the largest media companies in the world, he went nose to nose with all the premier broadcast networks. Risky and impulsive? Possibly. But it was likely to me that his hypomanic advantage gave him that "oomph"—the necessary drive, confidence, and vision to pull this megadeal off even when the naysayers had doubts. I've witnessed repeatedly that when you mix hypomania with great intellectual ability, you often get the classic energy, charm, and intuition that distinguishes many geniuses.

What about other celebrities such as real estate entrepreneur Donald Trump or even conservative talk show host Rush Limbaugh? Both have hyperthymic (see page 63) temperaments, and both probably have a propensity for beneficial hypomania, especially if you determine it by the traits of high energy, innovative brilliance, tremendous accomplishments, and ebullient charm. Because I have worked with many, I can usually spot these high achievers. Not only do they stand apart from the crowd, but they radiate extraordinary enthusiasm, charisma, and drive.

While these self-made celebrities may not be easy to live with (ask their families, former spouses, close friends, or co-workers), they have the very traits necessary to amass a great deal of fame, power, and wealth. A hypomanic Bipolar IIB may be described typically as driven or a "powerhouse of energy"; he or she may also be promiscuous and a fast talker. Many hypomanics are outspoken and often irritable to the point of being downright rude or abusive. They can also screw all of it up by impulsively dropping the ball or being discourteous to the wrong person.

Brad is an excellent illustration of the entrepreneurial spirit exhibited in Bipolar IIB. Extroverted and witty, Brad is the center of attention wherever he goes. He drives a BMW 760 sedan; his last car was a Mercedes Roadster, also the top of the line. Brad wants only the best in life, and if sales is one of the best ways to get rich, Brad was a superstar at a very young age. Now, at age 56, he and his third wife, 20 years his junior, bought a renovated English country cottage on the ocean in Long

Island's Easthampton. His two children live with his first wife in Los Angeles.

Brad owns two businesses and runs them from his three car phones. He keeps two lines busy most of the time, often well into the night; he calls the third line his backup. (His wife says he's surgically attached to his cell phones.) He was forced to get a driver, which allowed him to conduct business in his car, rather than waiting to get to one of his offices. Brad travels constantly and has been to Europe and Asia many times. Though his acquaintances think he's driven, I diagnosed him as Bipolar IIB. True, his friends and colleagues admire his energy and his enthusiasm, but sometimes they think Brad is somewhat out of control. Quite often, he comes up with ideas that seem over-the-top to them, like starting a joint manufacturing venture in Russia, when he had no prior experience, no Russian contacts, and did not even speak the language. His attorneys questioned and postponed the project. They had all they could do to talk him out of it, since crossing him could get them fired.

Brad is a sales genius because he is extremely perceptive about people and seems to sense almost immediately what they are thinking and feeling. He is always the center of a party, a meeting, an informal gathering. People are drawn to his energy and laughter. However, Brad can be his own worst enemy at times, particularly when he talks far too long at meetings. Brad speaks rapidly and is always spouting jokes or making rhymes or puns in his sales pitches. Sometimes people who don't know him well think he's doing cocaine or speed because his speech is so rapid-fire.

Brad's success is largely due to his hypomania. In contrast, if he had severe mania, he would hallucinate, become violent, perhaps end up in trouble with the law, or be hospitalized for psychotic behavior. With Brad, however, mania never becomes this severe. His mild mania means simply that he is often guilty of lapses in judgment, irritable, and sometimes driven to excess in spending and acquiring inconsequential "stuff."

At first, Brad came to see me unwillingly, at the insistence of his wife, who was about to leave him because of his drinking and his flirtatious nature with some of their friends and colleagues. She had read an article about Bipolar II disorder in *New York* magazine and was convinced that he had this problem.

Brad told me in the first office visit that he has never had a clinical depression that really kept him down. Although several times he had mild lows, he drank alcohol heavily for a couple of months until he felt spontaneously better. He mentioned that his father, a retired railroad executive, suffers from major depression and is being treated with antidepressants. His mother, who is "always in a good mood," as he said, is extremely active and driven, just like Brad. One of his sons, now in college, is taking antidepressants but makes superb grades and was voted president of the sophomore class. As I told Brad, this family history of mood disorders—and brilliant successes—is typical of many Bipolar IIB patients.

Exuberant and Confident

Perhaps by now you are wondering if any of the great political pundits may have been Bipolar IIB with a hypomanic temperament. As I originally wrote in *Moodswing,* so many politicians seem to exude charisma, enthusiasm, the gift of persuasion— and risky behavior. I do know that many great leaders exhibit the specific Bipolar II traits and are using the softer bipolar signs and symptoms to their greatest advantage. For example, when I think of an exuberant or hypomanic politician, former President Bill Clinton quickly comes to mind, particularly with his magnetic charm and high-spirited personality. I'm not saying that President Clinton is bipolar, since I have not consulted with him, but his garrulous and exuberant political style is definitely the hypomanic type.[4] Not only is the former president quick-thinking, verbose, and mildly elated, he is witty, talks fast, and is an ardent debater. Granted, he is obviously a risk-taker and a bit overly zealous when it comes to the opposite sex, but here again, risk-taking and overly zealous behaviors are two hypomanic qualities. Still, Clinton is highly confident with an infectious mood and hyperthymic temperament (see page 63) that make him extremely popular among millions both here and abroad.

The hypomanic drive of the Kennedy family is another example of how this exuberant state of mind can be transmitted from generation to generation. Almost all of the Kennedys are and have been energetic, quick-witted, extremely bright, loquacious, and outwardly confident, and I don't think these attributes were simply taught by their mothers and fathers. Rather, the hypomanic advantage is biochemical and genetic in origin: You either have it in the genes or you don't.

Looking back over history, the most charismatic president before John F. Kennedy was Theodore Roosevelt, the most hypomanic president ever to lead our nation and whose moods I described in my book *Moodswing.* Considering that one of Roosevelt's secretaries said that he wrote 150,000 letters during his governorship and presidency, I would say he was quite productive, with an active mind. Like many hypomanics, he was also said to be on the telephone or talking all the time, and he tried to cram his days with more than they could hold.

Abraham Lincoln also had hypomanic as well as depressive moods, both of which have been documented in numerous historical records and in my book *Moodswing.* Psychologists have long explained Lincoln's melancholic state, suggesting that a real or imagined loss must have preceded each of his "depressed" periods. We know that Lincoln had prolonged grief and deep depression after the death of his first love, Ann Rutledge, with accompanying symptoms of poor appetite and weight loss, sleeplessness, and suicidal threats. But while reactive depression from grief or a loss may resolve after weeks to a few months,

Lincoln's depression was far more integrated in his being and extended for many months after Ann's death, rendering Lincoln completely incapacitated. Curiously, after this depressive period, when Lincoln entered into social situations, he became the gregarious life of the party—talkative, jokey, and adaptive. Then, just as fast as he became the socializer, he went back into his moody, secretive state. Lincoln also used his "higher mood"—his hypomania—to his advantage as he leapt from an impoverished childhood in Illinois to the presidency of the United States.

It was only when one of these leaders extended themselves too far—like Lincoln did when he gave 20 speeches in 2 weeks and wound up physically and mentally exhausted—or used poor judgment—such as Roosevelt did during his presidency with lack of tact, constant friction and fighting, and always trying to impose his will on others—or fell into a depression that history had recorded evidence that many of our most captivating politicians were, in fact, masked cases of manic depression.

The psychodynamics of Winston Churchill are another case in point, and they have puzzled psychologists and psychiatrists for years. There is very little doubt that the former Prime Minister of England had a moody temperament, but his vitality and achievement were incredible. He survived until the age of 90; by 80 he had surmounted a heart attack, three bouts of pneumonia, two strokes, and two operations. He ate too much, drank too much, and smoked too much. Until he was 70, he rarely complained of fatigue, yet he had started life with considerable physical disadvantages, as had Teddy Roosevelt.

Today, Churchill would be described as cyclothymic (moody) or even manic-depressive. I would retrospectively diagnose Churchill as a classic Bipolar IIB. Of course, not every psychopharmacologist or psychiatrist would agree with this interpretation, or at least with the predominant emphasis I place on his tremendous achievements along with his moodswings. While I believe that medications may have alleviated his depressed moods, the stubborn "bulldog" would no doubt have insisted on brandy and soda instead, and history would not have been affected in the same way.

Highly Productive with an Antipathy toward Sleep

Perhaps one of the most reliable predictors of Bipolar IIB is the amount of sleep a person requires. Someone who sleeps less than 3 to 4 hours a night and functions well for long hours most probably is a hypomanic Bipolar IIB; he or she may have no complaints about insomnia. Now, if the average person gets 4 hours of sleep because of insomnia and drags through the next day just waiting to nap or get in bed, the chances are likely that he or she is not hypomanic. Rather, insomnia in this case may be a symptom of a general anxiety disorder or other psychiatric or medical disorder (see page 98). My hypomanic patients almost always show antipathy towards those who need to sleep. They consider sleep a waste of time and worry that they may be "missing out." These exceptional people thrive on very little sleep and use the nighttime hours to continue their intense path of high productivity. History reveals that the great inventor Thomas Edison (who was said to have a form of manic depression) slept only 3 to 4 hours at night, regarding sleep as unnecessary and a bother.

Eva, a popular jazz singer in New York City, told me during our first consultation, "I almost resent having to sleep at night because there are so many things I want to do. After singing a gig, I don't get home until well after midnight. I then take time to prepare a vegetarian meal, and then do my yoga positions before climbing into bed around 2:00 a.m."

Invariably, this 39-year-old jazz singer was wide awake at sunup each morning and could be seen walking her two black Labs down the sidewalks in Manhattan before 7:00 a.m. I have seen Eva at my office every year or so since her initial diagnosis of Bipolar II, but only when she falls low into a mild depression and needs medication to boost her mood. After a month or so, Eva's mood usually moderates and she functions normally, again getting by on very little sleep and a lot of activity. For the most part, this outstanding performer is extremely successful and energetic and has learned to live with her fairly consistent hypomanic mood, making it work for her.

Many of my Bipolar II patients, in fact, thrive on very little sleep, and most of the time, they report no adverse effect. Still, there are some patients who go for months with just a few hours of sleep each night and then suddenly their mood soars too high or falls low into the depths of depression. Take Mike, for example. Immediately after graduating from a college on the West Coast, this 31-year-old entrepreneur opened a restaurant on Manhattan's Upper West Side that became an internationally acclaimed four-star restaurant in no time and consistently received Best of New York awards for entrées and desserts. Mike worked 70- to 80-hour weeks for almost a decade to boost the restaurant's high standards. He began to receive regular national and international press and was asked by a national cable network to host a cooking show. Taping his show in the wee hours of the morning (the only time he was not at the restaurant), Mike was so energized, hyper-focused, and tireless that the TV crew wondered if he was on something illegal. He was extremely happy and on top of the world—getting by on just a few hours of sleep for weeks during the taping sessions—until he sunk low into a depression. It was at that time that he made an appointment to see me for medication.

I started Mike on a low dose of a mood stabilizer, along with an antidepressant to elevate his depressed mood. Within 2 weeks, his mood was within a normal range and he was back at his restaurant, working long hours and creating new recipes and menus.

I realized in talking with Mike that he was like so many high-achieving people with Bipolar IIB. He was able to capitalize on his extreme hypomanic periods to accomplish a great deal at a very young age. Yet, as with most individuals with Bipolar IIB, he extended too far and fell hard into a depression that necessitated medical treatment in order to lift his mood and allow him to function normally again.

Controlling but Cool

Some hypomanic personalities are what I call cool hypomanics. Rather than displaying the fast-talking, outwardly enthusiastic personality typical of most hypomanics, the cool hypomanic is restrained on the outside and may seem distant, emotionally in control, and calm. But the cool hypomanic is often a Bipolar IIB who simply keeps a very tight rein on his or her outward display of emotion while running a business empire, heading a major Wall Street law firm, or directing policy in a key government agency. His or her mind behind the external calm is whirling like a Jacuzzi.

You'd never know it to look at him, but Richard, the CEO of a major international publishing conglomerate based in New York City, is a textbook example of this "controlled" hypomanic. Richard travels regularly to London, Greece, Italy, France, Spain, and even Russia as he touches base with major subsidiaries of his company. He has been known to speak to senior management in five different countries over a period of 6 or 7 days and always looks like the quintessential corporate executive, even when jet lag is wreaking havoc on his physical and emotional stamina. Between his daily corporate meetings, his life is an almost unbroken succession of plane, train, or taxi rides, hurried snacks at widely irregular intervals, and 3- to 4-hour nights in foreign hotels with press conferences before breakfast or late at night when a new book is about to be released. Richard carries an unbelievable mental burden with the stressors of his ultra-fast-paced corporate life. Still, I have seen Richard let his guard down just a few times in the decade that I've treated him, and that was during a consultation in my office when he literally burst into tears while telling of all his responsibilities and how he felt too exhausted to tackle them.

Richard refuses to take a mood stabilizer. He confidently believes that he can manage his hectic lifestyle and myriad responsibilities without having a Bipolar II mood episode. So far, he has been able to stave off serious moodswings, but when I see him on television, he appears at times exhausted and even distracted. Perhaps he is able to control his moods with periodic breaks now and then, as he somehow manages to keep a strong, controlled presence that allows him to micromanage a successful multinational publishing company and be very convincing with the media.

Chatty and Persuasive

Mac's hypomanic ability to use three cell phones simultaneously almost cost him his life—literally. Mac, a 43-year-old salesperson by trade and all-around good guy, was known for keeping in touch with family, friends, colleagues, and clients twice daily. Most people thought he was just very friendly, persuasive, and chatty, but I suspected differently. Mac came to see me after nearly totaling his SUV on the New Jersey Turnpike during a rainstorm, because he was so preoccupied with using three cell phones. While holding for a call to his wife on one phone and listening to a message from his home office voice mail on the second phone, Mac was dialing out on the third phone and lost control of the wheel. His SUV slid and then veered directly onto the median, doing a 360 before flipping on its top. Other than a few bruises, Mac luckily was not injured, but he was in a state of shock and panic.

When we talked, I asked Mac if he had ever noticed any symptoms of depression. He looked at me in disbelief and said, "Are you kidding? I've had several weeks of depression lately that have robbed me of any energy. I've avoided my family, my friends, and my best clients, and I've lost income because of it."

Mac went on to describe the depressive times, saying he

hardly spoke to his wife or kids, and had a feeling of impending doom and hopelessness. "You can look at my corporate phone bills and see the times when I was feeling low—as the phone charges also dropped to nil."

The young salesman said that he was now sleeping 10 hours a night and eating excessively during these low times, harboring "a feeling of exhaustion that even additional sleep could not end." He required only around 4 hours of sleep when he was feeling high-spirited, and during his high-energy times, his sales records soared past his projections, helping to boost his superb income.

In my professional opinion, Mac was a classic case of Bipolar IIB. When hypomanic, he was extremely successful, closing a lot of deals and earning a high income. But Mac had the tendency to fall into periodic depressions where his energy and mood were low, and his ability to sell was stilted.

I explained the symptoms of pressured speech to Mac. His rapid-fire speaking pattern is evident when he talks uncontrollably. The pressured speech is sometimes manifested as extreme persuasiveness—a most useful trait in sales that helped Mac reach the top of his field and accumulate a small fortune at his age. When looking at the total picture with his history of recurrent depressions, Mac appeared to be a good candidate for medication to stabilize his Bipolar IIB moodswings without dampening his most successful hypomanic persuasiveness.

Intuitive and Captivating

Somehow, those with Bipolar IIB are wired to be around people. I call it PR metabolism. And when they are with people, they are usually in the limelight (if hypomanic). Like electrifying Pied Pipers, they are incredibly captivating, telling stories and jokes, patting people on the back, and making a big deal when you barely blink an eye.

Whether businesspeople or politicians, individuals with

Bipolar IIB can be very convincing with the people with whom they make deals. On the downside, I have experienced that many Bipolar IIB patients often use their charm and persuasiveness to control and manipulate their doctors or psychiatrists—often trying to avoid treatment, especially medication that they believe will dampen their hypomania.

Hypomanics are also more in touch with what is going on around them than most other people. For instance, the hypomanic tends to develop a sixth sense about gambling, because he may be open to grasping the thousands of small controlling factors that can win or lose a game. He is hyper-competent and jumps into every situation that he wants to control. For the hypomanic, knowledge is power. He is hyperperceptive, hyperaggressive, and hyperactive. He is tuned in to the games going on behind the games. He has a tremendous advantage so long as he doesn't overextend and start showing poor judgment by going too high.

Charming and Creative

I've already highlighted numerous Bipolar IIB traits such as risk-taking and being driven, highly productive, and energetic. There is still another positive characteristic of Bipolar IIB, and that is artistic creativity. Hypomanics, with their increased fluency and fluidity of thoughts, manifest highly creative traits that are consistent with those select men and women who gravitate toward the arts, particularly actors, composers, writers, poets, artists, and musicians. I originally described this link between creativity and bipolar illness in *Moodswing*.[3,5]

Many creative individuals, including some of Hollywood's greats—Ben Stiller, Jean-Claude Van Damme, Carrie Fisher, Patty Duke, Linda Hamilton, Jim Carrey, Margot Kidder, Tatum O'Neal—have openly professed in widely read magazines, as well as on talk shows, to having bipolar disorder. Some of television's best-known celebrities and actors, such as Mariette Hartley and *General Hospital*'s Maurice Bernard, have bipolar disorder and are now outspoken advocates, helping to educate others on this illness. Creative recording artist Sting has said in magazine interviews that he is manic-depressive, as have rappers DMX and MC Spice—and these are just a few recording artists who openly attest to having this disorder.

The humor that Jonathan Winters displayed is most likely related to his bipolar illness. After having a mental breakdown in 1960, Winters pulled back from the comedy nightclub gigs to spend more time at home. At that time, he concentrated on two other creative avenues, writing and painting, in both of which he excels. Winters went on to play Robin Williams's son Mearth on the television show *Mork and Mindy* and acted in other television roles.

Hanna, a 33-year-old gifted musician, composer, and graduate of New York's Juilliard School, described how her Bipolar IIB moodswings influence her creative flow and tremendous productivity.

"When my depressions began, I was working on several compositions and also playing harp at private gatherings. I was forcing myself to work. I couldn't think, much less create music. I reluctantly turned in one of my compositions during this time, and I can remember dreading the publisher's response. I felt like it was so horrible that I didn't want my name on it. I didn't want to hear it played. I couldn't sleep well at all, and I felt very, very alone.

"Finally, as time passed, the depression slowly lifted and turned into something else, which I didn't understand either, but I loved it! I became overly excited and filled with creative ideas. I slept very little, maybe 4 hours a night, and spent that extra time creating more music. I left my harp out in the living room and played it incessantly. There was no end to my love for this life as a musician. Instead of hating my compositions, I began to see that I was highly talented, and I continued to make changes until they were perfected. I suppose I was fairly ostentatious in my thoughts and speech, but I don't think I was annoying. I was definitely very active mentally and physically. I forgot about eating some days and lost about 30 pounds. I felt great! I just had so much to do and to create."

As Hanna and many others have experienced, during the times of Bipolar II depression, the tendency is to turn inward, brooding and questioning the creative work. Productivity also declines. But as I've witnessed with many creative Bipolar IIB patients, this low mood invariably boosts the artistic process as creativity breeds off the periodic mental anguish and then explodes into the energetic hypomanic expression, inner confidence, ideas, and productivity.

For Those with Bipolar II and Their Family Members

■ Just because an individual needs little sleep, is highly creative, and has an abundance of energy, it does *not* always indicate Bipolar II disorder. There are many men and women who need little sleep and who are superb leaders, brilliant entrepreneurs, and high achievers but who do not have moodswings, and who are not Bipolar IIB.

■ If you do have Bipolar II disorder, celebrate the highly adaptive, high-energy, hypomanic mood state described in this chapter that enables you to accomplish greatness. Take advantage of the productivity and nonstop ideas to rise to the top of your field. Get ample sleep each night to keep your mood in check so you don't soar too high and interrupt your success.

■ If you or a family member begins to extend too high with symptoms of needing less sleep, becoming haughty or irritable, or engaging in risky behaviors, seek medical treatment immediately with your mood specialist. There are specific medications discussed in chapter 8 and other interventions such as psychotherapy (see page 236) that can stop a moodswing from extending too far.

PART TWO

DIAGNOSIS AND TREATMENT OF BIPOLAR II

CHAPTER 7

THE BIPOLAR II CONSULTATION

We have come a long way in our ability to correctly diagnose and treat the softer moods on the bipolar disorder spectrum. As recently as the late 1950s, all manic-depressive illnesses were lumped together with schizophrenia, a serious mental illness sometimes referred to as a split personality, with symptoms of hallucinations, delusions, and incoherent speech. At that time, the treatment was the same no matter what the patient's mood: hydrotherapy, insulin coma therapy, electroshock treatment, and/or heavy tranquilizers. Today we realize that there are many signs and symptoms of bipolar disorder, and with an accurate diagnosis, most cases can be treated safely and effectively with medication—and, in some cases, without.

Recently I saw Christopher, a 34-year-old award-winning landscape architect, who had developed softer signs of bipolar disorder in his late twenties. Nothing serious, Christopher had thought at the time, and during the moodswings when his hyperalert mind would not stop racing or if he felt especially low, he would have a few drinks when he got home to relax. But the hypomania and depression intensified, as they usually do without mood-stabilizing treatment, and Christopher developed a tolerance for the alcohol. He began to drink more—the few drinks after work soon became a pint of Scotch every night to calm his mood. The alcohol gave him temporary relief, until he began to show some obvious signs of an addiction. For example, Christopher became very absentminded at work, missing client meetings, forgetting to complete corporate landscaping projects he had started, and neglecting to submit invoices for the projects he had completed. When clients began to seek landscaping services elsewhere, Christopher's employer put him on notice, giving him 30 days to seek help for his alcohol addiction or find a new job. About the same time, Christopher's wife had forgotten to restock his weekly supply of Scotch, and when Christopher found the liquor cabinet empty, he became outraged, screaming obscenities and hitting his wife. He then drove the family van to the liquor store and on the way home ran a stop sign and broadsided another car, sending a young mother and her toddler to the hospital with multiple injuries.

The next day, when Christopher arrived home from work, there was a note from his wife, saying she had left him and had taken their children to an undisclosed location, fearing for their safety. Christopher realized his moods and behaviors were out of control, and at the recommendation of his internist, he made an appointment to see me. After a long patient interview and physical exam with lab tests, I diagnosed Christopher with Bipolar II disorder and prescribed a small dose of lithium to help stabilize his highs and lows. I felt that the alcohol addiction was a very serious problem that needed immediate attention, and I convinced him to get involved in Alcoholics Anonymous, for the sake of his family, his career, and his own mental and physical well-being. Christopher's moods have stabilized, and he continues to check in every month for lab tests and talk therapy.

How unusual is Christopher's case? I do not know for sure, but it may be far more common than suspected, as Bipolar II disorder often coexists with alcohol or substance abuse addictions, which greatly complicate making an accurate diagnosis and prescribing the most effective treatment. For instance, about two-thirds of patients with Bipolar I and Bipolar II meet the diagnostic criteria for an addictive disorder,[1] and most psychiatrists fail to notice the very subtle and unspoken addiction patterns in the initial and subsequent interviews.

There are many factors to be considered before giving the diagnosis of Bipolar II disorder. For instance, I always question whether the patient is having moodswings from bipolar disorder or from a possible alcohol or drug addiction or even an undiagnosed illness. Is the person self-medicating with alcohol to soothe the mood, or is it just circumstantial? Is the alcohol causing the person to sleep poorly at night, or is it the bipolar disorder? The answers are not set in stone, and I always take a thorough patient history and have the internist who works in my office do a physical examination with laboratory tests in order to determine the underlying problem. All of us should keep Christopher's story in mind: Bipolar disorder is never treated effectively with alcohol or recreational drugs, and self-medicating the depression and hypomania usually complicates the problem and worsens the outcome.

People like Christopher who have bipolar disorder and a comorbid alcohol or drug abuse problem are five times more likely to commit suicide than those patients without the dual diagnosis. Bipolar II with comorbid substance abuse often presents as rapid-cycling or mixed states, with symptoms of extreme moodiness, short periods of elation, and deep depression. These feelings can last from hours to days to weeks. In a mixed state, the person would feel high and low, represented by irritability and paranoia. A trained psychiatrist should address these issues during the initial consultation and follow-up treatment.

In this chapter, I want to turn the focus from understanding the signs and symptoms of Bipolar II disorder to learning how the disorder is properly diagnosed and treated. Of course, there is no one laboratory test used to get a positive diagnosis. In addition, there is no single treatment that can cure Bipolar II disorder. But with an awareness of signs and symptoms and openness and honesty between patient and doctor, you can get the best outcome available for your mood disorder.

ACCURATE DIAGNOSIS IS CRUCIAL

An accurate diagnosis in Bipolar II is vital, as the diagnosis determines treatment. Yet in psychiatry, diagnosis can often be imprecise. Psychotic hallucinations, for example, can be a symptom of schizophrenia, which is notoriously difficult to treat, or of Bipolar I mania, which can be controlled with lithium. Unhappiness and feelings of emptiness and guilt can be certain characteristics of personality disorders or bipolar depression. The difference is major. If the diagnosis is depression, antidepressants or a mood stabilizer may help lift the mood. If the diagnosis is a personality disorder, the treatment involves many years of therapy and the prognosis is guarded. Thus, if a physician diagnoses a patient with a disease that he or she does not have, or for which there is no cure, then nothing will be done to help the patient. In this sense, whether a patient with bipolar disorder gets well—or not—may depend entirely upon the diagnosis. Finding an experienced psychiatrist or psychopharmacologist is critical because the diagnosis—along with the physician's knowledge of which drug to choose and in what dosage—ultimately determines the patient's outcome. If the presenting problem is so mild that the patient prefers to ride out the highs and lows without any medication or the usual course of treatment, then I would respect this decision and offer to follow the patient monthly on no medications.

Kimberly, a 37-year-old mother and homemaker, had lived with a persistent low mood for months before making an appointment to see me. After filling out the patient forms and a depression questionnaire, she gave me the following information:

"This past month I felt extremely sad and confused, emotionally exhausted, and completely lacking in physical or mental energy to the point where I would not even answer the phone, as I could not speak to anyone. I just wanted to sleep or lie in my bed holding my pillows. I wasn't interested in eating, shopping, or even being with my husband or children. My friends would stop by to check on me, but I would not answer the door. I wanted to be alone with my thoughts, as depressed as they were. Even though I felt so despondent and sad, I never cried. I mostly stared out in space, as if life was passing me by and I really couldn't care less.

"My sleep was greatly impaired for several months; it would take me 2 hours to finally fall asleep, and I have been waking up around 3:00 a.m. I have not been able to get back to sleep although I am exhausted and want to sleep all day. I have gained about 20 pounds in the past year, and although I don't eat much at meals, I snack all day. Food seems to give me some energy. I have considered suicide, but I don't think I'm at risk for following through with the act. Once I did take too many sleeping pills, but my husband saw me and rushed me to the emergency room for treatment."

Initially, Kimberly could not remember a time when she experienced hypomania, but then she recalled that there were several weeks each year, usually during the fall and spring, when she was "out of control with her spending and drinking and needed much less sleep." She did not realize it was hypomania at the time because it was such reprieve from her persistent low energy and depressed mood. Kimberly also shared that her mother was on an antidepressant, her brother had been an alcoholic for almost 8 years, and her mother's father had committed suicide when he was 40. I felt confident that Kimberly had Bipolar II disorder and prescribed a mood stabilizer with an antidepressant.

Kimberly is a perfect example of a Bipolar II patient who seeks treatment for the long and distressing bouts of depression without realizing that she also has periods of hypomania. Subsequently, many of these patients are given an incorrect diagnosis with the wrong treatment, as physicians unknowingly prescribe an antidepressant, which can lead to a rapid switch in mood and even to mania.

Ruling Out Physical Conditions

With today's high-tech medicine, we have become used to specialized and expensive laboratory tests to help the physician make a conclusive diagnosis. Most tests, however, are not very helpful in making the diagnosis of Bipolar II disorder. In fact, talking with the patient may be the most important diagnostic tool, as the person reports daily moods, behaviors, and lifestyle habits to the physician. While a physical examination will reveal a patient's overall state of health, the doctor must hear about specific signs and symptoms from the patient in order to effectively diagnose and treat Bipolar II.

There are some physical illnesses that frequently masquerade as a mood disorder. For example, systemic lupus erythematosus (lupus), thyroid disease, diabetes, multiple sclerosis, Lyme disease, epilepsy, syphilis, and HIV/AIDS can have signs and symptoms that often mimic those of Bipolar II, causing delayed treatment. Oftentimes, a simple blood test by a physician can eliminate these serious illnesses from consideration—or the blood work may indicate that the patient actually has a physical illness. For instance, a test for antinuclear antibody (ANA), an abnormal protein in the blood commonly found with lupus, can easily be done. If the doctor finds ANA, then he or she can do further investigation to see if the individual does, in fact, have this painful type of arthritis. A simple laboratory test can also reveal hyperthyroidism, which can mimic bipolar disorder with symptoms of irritability, mania, restlessness, and difficulty sleeping. Conversely, a blood test can also identify hypothyroidism, which can cause feelings of moodiness, depression, and overall fatigue. Because these bipolar-mimics are usually detected with lab work and are treatable or managed with medication, I always insist on obtaining blood chemistries as a key part of the initial patient consultation and physical exam.

In addition, numerous studies show the prevalence and clinical characteristics of anxiety disorders in those with Bipolar II, including generalized anxiety disorder, obsessive-compulsive disorder (OCD), panic disorder, phobic disorder, social anxiety disorder, and post-traumatic stress disorder (PTSD). If left untreated, each of these anxiety disorders can cause unnecessary suffering and impairment for the patient as well as his family.

Other problems often confound the proper diagnosis of Bipolar II, such as corticosteroids, which are medications commonly used to treat inflammatory diseases such as rheumatoid arthritis, asthma and allergy, ulcerative colitis, eczema, and psoriasis. These medications can cause episodes of depression and mania or hypomania that are sometimes mistaken for Bipolar II disorder.

Bipolar II or Medication?

A few months before I met 24-year-old Marla, she had been diagnosed by her internist as having rheumatoid arthritis and was put on high doses (60 milligrams per day) of prednisone, a corticosteroid medication, to decrease the inflammation in her joints. Marla told me she had battled moodswings within a week of starting the prednisone, initially feeling elated, energetic, and hyperalert, and then suffering a low, depressed mood that lasted several weeks. These two moods alternated with shorter 3-week bursts of what her doctor called mild mania and then depression. To treat her inflammatory arthritis, Marla's internist kept her on the high dose of prednisone, but he also gave her a mood-stabilizing medication to counter the moodswings, along with an antidepressant for the depression and a heavy sedative so she could sleep at night. When the young woman walked into my office that first time, she looked like a zombie. Accompanied by her parents, who were desperate to get her help, Marla said she was virtually homebound because her mood was so unstable and the medications kept her from functioning normally.

As we talked, I learned more about Marla's family and her background. There was no history of psychiatric illness or problems such as alcohol or substance abuse in her family, and she had never suffered with depression or hypomania before taking this medication. The young woman had an outstanding personal history of achievement and a successful academic career. In fact, she had finished her undergraduate requirements in just 3 years and was then accepted into the master's of science in mathematics program at Columbia.

About the same time that she started the graduate program, she started having tremendous joint pain, daily fatigue, and sudden weight loss and saw a rheumatologist for an evaluation. After doing a physical exam and performing lab tests, the doctor diagnosed her with rheumatoid or inflammatory arthritis and prescribed prednisone.

At first, the prednisone made Marla feel elated, which is common with this type of therapy, even in individuals with past or current symptoms of depression. Not only was the joint pain lessened, but her mood and energy level were greatly elevated. Whereas before she was getting 8 or 9 hours of sleep a night, she now was getting by on less than 5 hours of sleep and was not missing it at all. Marla began to stay up all hours of the night reading her coursework and working on papers that were not due until the end of the semester. Then after about 2 weeks, Marla felt so elated that she left the books and started to go out at night with fellow classmates, often spending the night with several young men she barely knew from school. She began dressing in a flamboyant way with tight clothes and even a naval piercing—all vastly different from her previous conservative appearance.

During the months that followed, Marla fell into several cyclical mood and behavioral swings. As long as she stayed on the massive doses of prednisone, her rheumatoid arthritis stayed in remission. She had no pain and tremendous energy. But she felt like the medication was now causing her to feel too high and then too low, as she dove into brief periods of depression where she could barely get out of bed and did not want to leave her bedroom. Finally, she dropped out of the prestigious graduate school program for the semester and spent her days sleeping or watching soap operas at her parents' home.

Marla exhibited symptoms of both hypomania and depression. Yet these symptoms abated each time her rheumatologist reduced the amount of prednisone she was taking for her illness. When the medication dosage was lowered, her joint pain and fatigue increased to the point where she had to go on higher doses of prednisone again. When her doctor added the sedatives to "calm her mood," she felt like a zombie.

I explained to Marla the limited data on prednisone that suggests symptoms of hypomania, mania, depression, and even acute psychosis are common during therapy, usually in doses higher than 40 milligrams per day. Typically, the mood symptoms are dose dependent with corticosteroid therapy and can begin during the first few weeks of treatment, just as Marla had experienced, although some patients never experience wide moodswings. Some findings indicate that these mood and cognitive changes are reversible side effects, meaning that once patients go off the corticosteroid, they will return to their normal mood state—as was Marla's experience. While a few studies indicate that the antipsychotic drug Zyprexa (olanzapine) is well tolerated and useful for mood disturbances associated with corticosteroid therapy, I felt that Marla and I should work with her rheumatologist to see if another medication, along with a reduced dose of prednisone, could treat her inflammatory arthritis.

Marla is now taking a small dose of prednisone along with another immunosuppressant drug to keep her rheumatoid arthritis in remission. Her mood is back to normal with neither high nor low moodswings, and she has returned to her graduate program at Columbia. She continues to see her rheumatologist monthly to make sure her arthritic condition is managed, but she has no further need to check in with me.

I give the example of Marla and her corticosteroid-induced hypomania and depression to show how a misdiagnosis of bipolar disorder is not uncommon among patients and physicians today. Yet with an incorrect diagnosis, there is great suffering as treatment is ineffective or may even worsen the initial condition. When doctors treat misdiagnosis and moodswings improperly, the patient's risk of attempting suicide is increased. Some patients, like Marla, simply need a few medication adjustments to resolve their moodswings that mimic those of bipolar disorder.

NBC-TV newswoman Jane Pauley also experienced the side effects of medication-induced hypomania and depression when she was treated with steroids for a case of hives. In her book *Skywriting,* Pauley revealed that she has bipolar disorder. When she was first prescribed steroids, she initially experienced hypomania. However, she became depressed on the second administration of the steroids, so her doctor prescribed a low-dose antidepressant. Pauley then experienced agitation and rapid cycling of moods until she was hospitalized and her moodswings were stabilized on lithium. Left untreated, bipolar moodswings can increase in frequency over time and may then become resistant to treatment altogether.

Assessing the Risk of Moodswings

While emotions play a role in many illnesses, with Bipolar II, openly assessing mood on a daily basis can be most helpful in making an accurate diagnosis and receiving the best and most effective treatment with the fewest side effects.

Review the questionnaires that follow and fill in each item. Do not take too long thinking about the answer, as I have found the immediate reaction is usually more accurate than a long, thought-out response. While these two questionnaires cannot give you a complete diagnosis, they can prompt you to share the results with your doctor and discuss possible problems with depression and/or hypomania.

Depression Questionnaire

YES	NO	
		1. Has your predominant mood been:
		a. Mainly anxious
		b. Mainly angry
		c. Mainly apathetic
		d. Loss of interest
		e. Mainly depressed
		f. Anxious and depressed
		g. Mixed-euphoric
		h. Mainly euphoric/expansive
		i. Mainly angry/paranoid
		j. Mainly irritable
		k. Mixed with depression
		2. Did you have any of the following symptoms during the past week?
		a. Depressed mood most of the day nearly every day; crying for no reason
		b. Markedly diminished interest/pleasure in most activities
		c. Significant weight loss/gain (more than 5% in a month)
		d. Decrease in appetite nearly every day
		e. Feeling slowed down/fatigued/depleted of energy every day
		f. Feeling worthless, helpless, hopeless, or excessive guilt every day
		g. Recurrent thoughts of death, thoughts that life is not worth living, or thoughts of suicide
		h. Difficulty in concentration/inability to think or stay focused, indecisiveness nearly every day
		3. Have you had any of the following anxious/nervous symptoms in the past 6 months?

(continued)

		a. Worry and apprehension about a number of events nearly every day and find these feelings difficult to control
		b. Restlessness or feeling keyed up or on edge
		c. Easily fatigued or irritable
		d. Muscle tension/tightness in the back, neck, or shoulders
		e. Sleep disturbance (difficulty in falling or staying asleep or restless, unsatisfying sleep)
		f. Moderate to severe difficulty in social and occupational functions
		4. In the past week have you been feeling elated, hypomanic, or manic?
		5. Have you been very irritable, angry, easily annoyed?
		6. In the past week have you had any of the following symptoms:
		a. Were you more active than usual socially, at home or at work? More sexually active? More physically restless (unable to sit still)?
		b. Were you more talkative than usual or did you feel pressured to keep on talking?
		c. Did you feel you were a very important person, had special powers, plans, talents, or abilities?
		d. Did you do anything foolish that could have gotten you into trouble like buying things, business investments, sexual indiscretions, reckless driving?
		e. Did you have trouble concentrating on what was going on because your attention kept jumping to unimportant things around you?
		f. Did you need less sleep than usual for 3 days or more? If YES, specify:
		No sleep at all
		Less than 3 hours
		Between 3–6 hours
		g. Did your thoughts race or did you talk so fast that it was difficult for people to follow what you were saying?

Mood Disorder Questionnaire

YES	NO	
		1. Has there ever been a period of time when you were not your usual self and:
		a. You felt so good or so hyper that other people thought you were not your normal self or you were so hyper that you got into trouble?
		b. You were so irritable that you shouted at people or started fights or arguments?
		c. You felt much more self-confident than usual?
		d. You got much less sleep than usual and found you didn't really miss it?
		e. You were much more talkative or spoke faster than usual?
		f. Thoughts raced through your head or you couldn't slow your mind down?
		g. You were so easily distracted by things around you that you had trouble concentrating or staying on track?
		h. You had much more energy than usual?
		i. You were much more active or did many more things than usual?
		j. You were much more social or outgoing than usual, for example, you telephoned friends in the middle of the night?
		k. You were much more interested in sex than usual?
		l. You did things that were unusual for you or that other people might have thought were excessive, foolish, or risky?
		m. Spending money got you or your family into trouble?
		2. If you checked YES to more than one of the above, have several of these ever happened during the same period of time?
		3. How much of a problem did any of these cause you—like being unable to work; having family, money, or legal troubles; getting into arguments or fights? (Please select one of the following.)
		No problem
		Minor problem
		Moderate problem
		Serious problem

BE YOUR OWN MENTAL HEALTH ADVOCATE

After taking the questionnaires on pages 167 to 169, you may begin to wonder if you have signs of Bipolar II. Forty-one-year-old Gary took the two tests when he first came to see me and realized that he had experienced signs of hypomania and depression over the past few years. While his mood had seemed normal at the time, he felt unusually excitable and was having difficulty sleeping more than a few hours at night and staying focused on his music. He went ahead and made an appointment with his primary care physician for a physical examination. Gary was then referred to my office for a consultation. I diagnosed this accomplished musician, who played French horn in a major symphony orchestra, as having Bipolar II and put him on a mood stabilizer with a low dose of an antidepressant. Today, Gary comes in monthly for a brief visit to check his blood levels of medication and to discuss any recurrent symptoms, mood-swings, or side effects of the medications.

While your doctor is your medical advocate, it is important to become your own mental health advocate to get the best diagnosis and treatment. This means making your health a priority and even getting a second opinion, if necessary, to ensure that your diagnosis is accurate and your treatment is most effective.

Choose a Specialist

Because of the complex nature of this increasingly common disorder—and the fact that each patient is different—it is imperative that you seek an accurate diagnosis and effective treatment from a board-certified physician who can be trusted to take responsibility for your overall mental health. Board certified means that the doctor has passed a standard examination given by the national governing board in that specialty. You should look for a person who is trained in psychiatry or psychopharmacology.

If you are seeking a well-qualified psychiatrist, you might check with the chairperson's office at the nearest major university's department of psychiatry. From there, you can get a list of qualified specialists or a referral to the university medical center to see one of the doctors on campus. Many faculty members affiliated with a medical school's department of psychiatry see private patients and work at low-cost university clinics as well. These physicians can also refer patients to a private practice physician.

Because of managed care, finding the right person to diagnose and treat Bipolar II disorder properly and cost-effectively is not always easy. For those with an HMO, a "gatekeeper" or primary care physician must make the referral to a psychiatrist specializing in psychopharmacology. Carefully read the policy manual to understand the specific rules and to see if a specialist is covered. Then select a physician whom you can trust to know your personal and family medical history and take responsibility for your health care.

Perhaps one of the most important steps to take when selecting a psychiatrist/psychopharmacologist is to know yourself, including your personal likes and dislikes. Do you feel more comfortable with a man or woman? Should your psychiatrist be older than you, the same age, or younger? Do you have a preference as to educational background? Should the doctor's office be near your home or work? Does the doctor see patients after hours, in case of emergency? These questions are important to consider when making your selection and initial appointment to ensure that you will feel comfortable talking with the physician and that you will keep regular appointments for ongoing therapy and lab work, if necessary.

Write Down Concerns and Seek Answers

Before your appointment with the psychiatrist, write down a list of concerns you may have about Bipolar II disorder and specific symptoms you need help with. I recommend taking the two questionnaires from this chapter with you to the appointment to help the doctor in assessing your moodswings. It is also helpful to get an in-depth family history from relatives before meeting with your doctor. So many times, this crucial information is key in making an accurate diagnosis and prescribing effective treatment.

Before your visit, consider and record the following:

- Your mental and physical health concerns
- Symptoms you've noticed
- Unusual behaviors you've had
- Past illnesses (both physical and mental)
- Your family history of mental illness (manic depression, major or clinical depression, anxiety disorders, personality disorders, alcohol and substance abuse, suicide, arrests, and even outstanding achievement, as I discussed beginning on page 66)
- Medications you are taking now and have taken in the past, including prescribed and over-the-counter; unusual side effects of medications you are taking or have taken
- Natural dietary supplements or herbs you are taking
- Your lifestyle habits (exercise, diet, smoking, caffeine and alcohol consumption, drugs such as marijuana, cocaine, amphetamines, tranquilizers)
- Your sleep habits
- Causes of stress in your life (marriage, work, social)
- Questions you have about Bipolar II disorder

Evaluate Your Moods and Behavior

In my experience, there is an art to identifying and treating the elated and energetic patient with Bipolar IIB who feels extraordinarily well in his or her mild hypomanic phase. As stated, many of these men and women use their energy positively, and they are high achievers whose moodswings become a problem usually in the down phase. But when they arrive in the office of the psychiatrist or primary care physician complaining of depression, the doctor may overlook a subtle history of hypomanic symptoms. Usually the patient responds to the doctor with denial and resistance, so a spouse, another family member, or a friend is often the one to supply the necessary information to the doctor or psychiatrist during the first interview to help establish the correct diagnosis.

In addition to reviewing your own detailed family history before your appointment, examine your own past mood episodes, behaviors, and achievements and record these. Do not overlook periods of high energy and accomplishment. If necessary, ask your spouse or another close family member or friend, as these periods may be clues of Bipolar II disorder. The diagnosis of bipolar illness in the *DSM-IV* completely overlooks the benefits of the high periods present in some patients' mood cycles. Thus, a great leader such as Winston Churchill would simply be labeled manic-depressive, implying a defect only, this failing to include his extremely gifted beneficial side. A wife, husband, or friend will remember times of high functioning that the depressed patient, in his lethargy, sadness, or despair, cannot or does not want to recall. In a depressed state, the patient feels useless and no good. Without additional input, the doctor can easily misdiagnose the disorder as recurrent major depression or as dysthymia (see page 50). With an incorrect diagnosis, the physician or psychiatrist often prescribes wrong and ineffective medication such as an antidepressant alone, which may trigger hypomanic behavior and rapid-cycling, which may ultimately lead to suicidal thoughts in misdiagnosed individuals.

Review Your Medications and Supplements

Bring your medications and any nutritional supplements you may be taking along with you on your first visit to see the doctor. Your doctor will let you know which ones are safe to continue using—depending on an analysis of the drugs or supplements along with your diagnosis and new medications.

DR. FIEVE'S MULTIPHASE DIAGNOSIS/ TREATMENT APPROACH

In my New York practice, I employ a multiphase diagnosis/treatment process, which consists of a detailed psychiatric diagnostic evaluation and interview, a physical examination, biochemical and screening tests, and regular monitoring of the patient to ensure the treatment is working at an optimum level. I also prescribe psychotherapy for many of my patients with Bipolar II and consider this an essential part of the medical protocol.

Phase 1: Initial Evaluation and Diagnosis

The first step in the Bipolar II disorder diagnosis and treatment process involves a preliminary patient medical and psychiatric evaluation and a review of the standard diagnostic criteria for Bipolar II as presented in the *DSM-IV*.

Psychiatric history and evaluation. The psychiatric history and evaluation are essential, especially given the extensive differential possibilities that are likely when the patient presents with symptoms of depression, sleeplessness, inability to concentrate or focus, restlessness, increased or decreased energy, weight and appetite changes, sexual changes, and hypomania or mania.

When a patient says he feels "low, lifeless, and without hope," it is difficult to say where he fits on the manic-depressive spectrum. To treat him effectively, the doctor must know more about the patient and his family. Likewise, in my practice, if a patient comes into the office all revved up, is talking fast, and feels overconfident and haughty, I cannot precisely and immediately say where he or she fits on the bipolar spectrum. After taking the patient's chief complaint, present illness, personal history, past history, and family history and reviewing a recent physical examination, I usually make the differential diagnosis that allows me to eliminate other serious problems that might be causing the symptoms and, thus, come up with Bipolar II disorder or another diagnosis, depending on the case. By then, I will have eliminated the illnesses that usually confound this diagnosis, such as Bipolar I, schizophrenia, schizo-affective disorder, major depression, dysthymia, generalized anxiety disorder, personality disorder, attention-deficit/hyperactivity disorder, and drug and alcohol abuse, among others.

The doctor/patient interview. Although some clinicians may feel more comfortable using predetermined interview questions, such as those on pages 167 to 169, they should be aware that standard tests are often insensitive to hypomanic symptoms. In trying to avoid this, I begin my consultation with questions such as the following:

1. Can you tell me what sort of symptoms are bothering you, when did they begin, and how much are they disabling your present life at home, at work, or socially?
2. If you had your way, can you prioritize the specific moods in your own life that you would like me to help you with, eliminate, or keep?
3. If the patient is complaining of a lot of anxiety as well as depression: If I was able to eliminate only one of these two major complaints—anxiety or depression—which one would you want me to eliminate?
4. How depressed have you been (mild, moderate, severe)?

At this point in the discussion, I turn to the specific criteria listed in the *DSM-IV*, as noted in chapter 2, to evaluate the patient's severity of hypomania or depression. I also take a detailed history of each hypomanic, manic, or depressive episode over the patient's lifetime, including symptoms, duration, severity, and treatment. When the number of episodes starts increasing beyond four or five, I have to structure the interview in a different way. For example, if there are multiple episodes of depression, I ask the patient to estimate the amount of time over 10 to 20 years that he has been in a depressive, manic, hypomanic, or normal mood state. After reviewing the responses to these questions, the family history, and the physical exam, I can then, confidently, make a correct diagnosis.

Phase 2: Physical Examination and Laboratory Testing

The second phase in the multiphase diagnosis/treatment approach entails doing the physical examination and conducting all relevant lab tests, listing all drugs the patient may be currently taking or has taken in the past, and obtaining the measures of these drugs in the body, using blood and urine tests (if necessary). Based on the obtained laboratory results from phase 2, along with the *DSM-IV* diagnosis as determined in phase 1, I usually begin medication and initiate treatment procedures as well as cognitive psychotherapy with Dr. Patrick Murphy, the associate psychologist in my New York practice.

Physical examination. Perhaps I am one of few psychopharmacologists who insist on an electrocardiogram (ECG) and blood and urine testing with the physical examination. At first, many new patients resist this policy, but then they begin to appreciate the fact that a psychiatrist who is also interested in their physical health and overall well-being, as well as their psychological state, is to be trusted. In addition, patients who are on lithium for years for bipolar treatment are at greater risk of thyroid or kidney problems. Detecting and managing a beginning thyroid or kidney problem before it escalates allows the doctor to prevent a later serious illness.

In performing the patient physical examination, the medical doctor will primarily focus on the neurologic and endocrine systems and try to identify major health concerns that may be contributing to symptoms of depression or hypomania. For example, hypothyroidism is the most common medical condition associated with depressive symptoms. Many central nervous system illnesses and injuries, including syphilis, central nervous system tumors, multiple sclerosis, stroke, various cancers (pancreas, prostate, breast), and head trauma are also accompanied by a secondary diagnosis of depression. Hyperthyroidism, Cushing's disease, hyperparathyroidism, and corticosteroid medications (as discussed earlier in this chapter) can also induce hypomania and depression. Certain drugs, including illegal steroids, amphetamines, and over-the-counter appetite suppressants, may cause outbursts of mania or hypomania or precipitate depression upon withdrawal.

Screening tests. Screening tests may vary, depending on your age, gender, symptoms, and health history. I use any or all of the following routine screening tests with the initial and annual physical examinations.

- Blood pressure monitoring
- Routine blood chemistries
- An initial and yearly routine electrocardiogram (ECG)
- Urine analysis (initial screening; periodic testing for comorbid drug abuse)
- Prostate-specific antigen (PSA) test for prostate cancer (men over 40 or with a family history of cancer)
- Other cancer screening tests (If these tests come back positive, I offer a referral to other physicians who are specialists in specific fields.)
- Chest x-ray (I order this test only if the patient has not had a chest x-ray in 3 to 4 years or has pulmonary symptoms.)

Patients who come to my office are required to have a blood chemistry profile that measures, among other substances, the level of thyroid hormones. Because an amount below the normal range may be sufficient in itself, in some cases, to cause depression, patients with underactive thyroids may need to take thyroid hormone medication. If the depression has not begun to disappear on thyroid hormone alone, after 2 to 8 weeks, I prescribe a trial of an antidepressant. However, if patients are already in a major depression superimposed on the hypothyroidism, which is referred to as a double depression, they will need an antidepressant as well as the thyroid hormone.

Other standard tests included in the initial physical examination are blood tests to check electrolytes, liver function, and kidney function. Because the kidneys and liver are responsible for the elimination of bipolar medications, impairment of either of these two organs may cause the drugs to accumulate in the body. For this reason, patients with renal disease, as evidenced by high BUN (blood urea nitrogen) or serum creatinine, including those undergoing hemodialysis, may have to be treated with smaller dosages of the drug, or an alternative drug altogether. Annual monitoring with kidney function tests is required for all lithium patients, and sometimes a nephrologist (an internist who specializes in the diagnosis and treatment of kidney disease) is consulted if kidney problems arise. If you have severe kidney or liver disease, do not take lithium or anticonvulsant drugs. Talk with your doctor about other treatment modalities for your Bipolar II disorder.

High-tech neuro-imaging. Some high-technology neuro-imaging tests such as positron emission tomography (PET scan or PET imaging), magnetic resonance imaging (MRI), and single proton emission computed tomography (SPECT) may offer new hope for making more specific psychiatric diagnoses and clarifying how the body metabolizes a specific drug the patient is being given for treatment.[2] Already researchers are mapping out specific PET and SPECT brain scan patterns for bipolar disorder, schizophrenia, drug abuse, and alcoholism. Neuro-imaging techniques are increasingly used to study the regional pharmacokinetics of medications, including lithium and anticonvulsants, to understand the specific changes in neurotransmission that go along with disease remission. In that light, neuro-imaging may help doctors arrive at a safe and therapeutic dose of a *specific* drug needed for a *specific* patient with a *specific* condition . . . such as Bipolar II disorder.

Phase 3: Weekly to Monthly Monitoring

Depending on the prescribed medication and the patient's symptoms, I see the patient weekly, biweekly, or monthly in the third phase. On each visit, I assess the patient's degree of improvement in mood and behavior and any side effects against what is usual for patients on that particular medication, discuss whether or not the patient is experiencing suicidal ideas, and monitor blood levels of the drug. There are optimal therapeutic levels of lithium and other drugs that must be achieved in order for the mood to be stabilized. Some medications such as lithium must be monitored continually, as they can become toxic. After the blood tests, which are drawn right in my office, are completed and I have received the blood medication levels, I readjust dosages of the medications to further improve the response and decrease side effects when indicated. In some cases, I have to change medications when, after 4 to 6 weeks, the patient reports minimum or no response, or if the medication's side effects are intolerable.

Phase 4: Psychotherapy

About 50 percent or more of my Bipolar II patients also have coexisting interpersonal problems in their marriages, at work, or within their social lives. I recommend that these patients start regular cognitive psychotherapy sessions, which are further discussed in chapter 10. At my private practice, psychotherapy sessions are performed by one of my associate psychologists; if your psychiatrist does not have a referring psychologist, it is important that he or she talk regularly with the psychologist you select and share notes regarding moodswings, treatment, and other concerns. Patients who undergo psychotherapy as well as psychopharmacology treatment know that their psychologist and I discuss their condition on a weekly basis. That communication is of extreme importance in the patient's overall education and treatment.

For Those with Bipolar II and Their Family Members

- The initial consultation with a psychiatrist or psychopharmacologist can be confusing. I can tell by the looks on my patients' faces that they are frightened by what they are feeling—the depressive and hypomanic signs and symptoms—as well as the impending psychiatric and laboratory test results and possible diagnosis. I find it most helpful when patients bring a family member or close friend with them for the initial appointment. Taking someone with you can ease your anxiety, so you feel confident in telling the doctor exactly how you feel. Also, many times family members are more aware of moodswings than the patient is and can share this crucial information with the doctor for a more accurate diagnosis.

- Keep in mind that depending on your mood, treatment for Bipolar II may be as simple as keeping a watchful eye on the symptoms, with no medications prescribed at all. In some cases of mild hypomania, I believe that a low-keyed spouse or quiet, laid-back close friend is often the equivalent of a mood-modulating medication.

- If your doctor diagnoses you with Bipolar II disorder and prescribes an antidepressant or mood stabilizer to regulate the extreme highs and lows, it is imperative to check in with the doctor periodically to make sure the symptoms are well managed and the dosage is correct. Write down on paper any unusual feelings you are having and share this information with your doctor at the visit. Your doctor only knows what you say, so try not to hold back much-needed feedback.

- If your moodswings are more severe, your doctor may prescribe a "cocktail" of several medications to stabilize the mood and ask you to come in weekly or biweekly to test blood levels of the medications. To keep your mood balanced and to give you the highest quality of life, it's vital to listen to the doctor and comply with this simple request. As the medications work to modulate your mood, the visits to your doctor will be less frequent.

CHAPTER 8

MODULATING MOODS

The concept of bipolar disorder's moodswings is so entwined in the public's consciousness that many people today casually use the word *manic* to describe themselves after drinking two cups of coffee or a "hyper" friend who might be overly energetic or chatty. The term *depressed* is carelessly used when you can't zip your new jeans or it is time to mail the IRS payment. The problem is that many people with Bipolar II disorder who are hypomanic or depressed often accept these feelings as being their normal mood, when, in fact, they could have optimum emotional health with a proper psychiatric diagnosis and effective treatment.

In many cases, the moodswings of Bipolar II are often pleasurable and do not resolve without medication or other treatment. Feeling hypomanic is not the same as having an abundance of energy and ideas or feeling exceptionally happy one day. Being depressed is not a temporary low mood that happens when you gain 10 pounds over the holidays or a long-awaited vacation is postponed. Likewise, the medications used for Bipolar II disorder are not used for these transitory elated or down feelings. The vicissitudes of daily life are part of our normal range of emotions.

On the other hand, when a patient tells me his or her hypomanic mood has lasted for 4 or more days or if the mood extends too far and is accompanied by a number of *DSM-IV* symptoms (see page 49), I can usually make an accurate diagnosis and prescribe the most effective mood-modulating medication that allows the person to return to a normal mood within days to weeks. Likewise, if the patient tells of having a depressed mood that lasts for more than a few weeks and is accompanied by symptoms outlined in the *DSM-IV* (see pages 51 and 55), I can diagnose the major depression or dysthymia and prescribe the appropriate medication to give the patient much-needed relief from the low mood.

In this chapter I will address the importance of specific medications in modulating mood and also explain why sometimes a patient might need two drugs to keep moods stable. With a greater understanding of moodswings from part one of this book and of how the cycles of depression and hypomania can literally rule—and sometimes even ruin—your life, you can ask your doctor about the medications discussed in this chapter and see if one might help your situation or that of a loved one.

MURIEL'S MOODS

For those with Bipolar II, the correct medications make all the difference in normalizing moodswings and giving back a normal quality of life. I consulted with a prominent Manhattan magazine publisher a few years ago after she had attempted to "self-medicate" her months of major depression and almost lost her life. This 49-year-old woman's frank admission of how she coped with and self-treated her moodswings is both typical and revealing:

"Three or four Xanax before work. Two Valium before bedtime. A weekend in Vegas. A double Scotch at breakfast; another at lunch. Two divorces and two remarriages. Deadlines that made me scream at loyal employees. A weekend flight to Paris.

More Scotch. Another marriage and divorce. An entire new wardrobe. Move in with my new boyfriend. A handful of 'dexies.' Twenty-three hours of sleep, and more 'dexies.'"

When I first met Muriel, she had just been discharged from the psychiatric unit after having taken a drug overdose when her boyfriend said he was leaving her for a younger woman. For years, this brilliant and very attractive woman had suffered needlessly with the major depression so common with Bipolar II disorder but was too proud to seek medical treatment. During our initial consultation, Muriel said that she thought the miserable down periods would vanish forever if she could only try to stay happy and "upbeat." She therefore tried to find happiness—spending thousands of dollars each month on whims, changing live-in lovers with the seasons, and taking handfuls of pills with alcohol. Usually, by the time the depression did resolve, she was hypomanic, which made her ebullient, enthusiastic, and highly effective as a publisher and in her relationships. It was during the hypomanic times that she acquired smaller publications, came up with exciting campaigns to increase her target audience, and made the opposite sex fall in love with her again and again. She then quickly forgot the melancholic and dejected mood that had haunted her the previous weeks to months until it started to drag her down again.

As Muriel and I talked and began to unpeel the many layers of scars she wore from her years of untreated depression, I explained that the very things she was using to self-medicate the blues—mainly drugs and alcohol—actually deepen depression. As I explained in chapter 5, self-medicating with a drug or alcohol addiction is a comorbid problem for many bipolar patients and can lead to suicide. Perhaps what bothered me the most about Muriel is that she had cheated herself in not seeking proper treatment for her moodswings. In almost all cases of Bipolar II disorder, there are excellent treatments to control the cyclic aspect of depression or hypomania—and most drugs that we use today have few harmful side effects. If one drug has unwanted side effects, a knowledgeable psychiatrist or psychopharmacologist can try another until the patient finds the medication that works best.

While I cannot guarantee that the medications discussed in this chapter will solve every person's moodswings, it is important to understand the categories of treatment—and specific medications—that are working for many with Bipolar II as part of a successful management and prevention program.

After you have read this entire chapter, call and talk to your doctor about the medications you are taking to see if they are the most effective ones for your diagnosis with the fewest side effects possible. Working closely with your psychiatrist or psychopharmacologist, you should be able to find the best treatment with the fewest side effects that meets your particular mood needs and allows you to live an active and meaningful life.

LITHIUM AND THE AGE OF PSYCHOPHARMACOLOGY

Lithium is one of the oldest and least expensive of the mood-stabilizing drugs for bipolar disorder, and most all of the world's bipolar experts still think it is the best. This naturally occurring salt, a simple white powder found in mineral water and rock, and in smaller amounts in plant and animal tissue, is administered as a salt available under the generic names of lithium carbonate and lithium citrate. Manufacturers of lithium also assign "trade names" to their products, such as Eskalith, Lithobid, Lithane, Lithonate, Lithotabs, Cibalith-S, and others. Lithium is available in capsule, tablet, or liquid form.

Lithium as a Mood Stabilizer

GENERIC NAME	TRADE NAME
Lithium carbonate	Eskalith, Lithane, Lithobid
Lithium citrate	Cibalith-S (liquid)

The serendipitous discovery of lithium as a treatment for bipolar disorder was groundbreaking and consequently opened doors to further discoveries over the next 5 decades. In 1949, Australian psychiatrist John Cade, MD, senior medical officer in an Australian hospital, discovered the anti-manic effects of lithium quite by accident. Years later, when Dr. Cade visited me in New York City, he explained that while trying to figure out what might be wrong in the brains of patients with manic-depressive illness, he wondered whether a soluble form of urea might have therapeutic value.

Knowing that the poisonous waste of the kidneys comes out in the form of urea, Dr. Cade hypothesized that urine contained a toxin specific to manic depression. So, he thought: "Let's see if my idea is right—the urine of manics is poisoned." Dr. Cade extracted the urea from the urine. To make it soluble, he added lithium to it quite by accident. He theorized that if pigs injected with the urea became agitated, that would prove his theory. Instead, they became lethargic—from the lithium, thus, leading to his discovery.

Dr. Cade was thrilled with this finding and began administering lithium to manic patients with tremendous results, as the manic excitement was alleviated without heavy sedation.

A major turning point in the history of lithium occurred in 1954, when Danish researcher Mogens Schou, MD, and colleagues published their first double-blind study of lithium in mania, initiating Dr. Schou's lifelong passionate pursuit of lithium research and teaching. Dr. Schou personally disseminated the evolving information on lithium with his prolific writings and lecturing over the next 40 years, by traveling from country to country and stimulating thousands of investigators and clinicians on all continents worldwide. Dr. Schou has been the single most important psychiatrist in the history of lithium therapy, following Dr. Cade's discovery.

It seemed only natural then that in the late 1950s, while I was a resident-in-charge of the acute psychiatric service at the

New York State Psychiatric Institute, we began hearing about the promising results from Australia and Denmark about the use of lithium carbonate in treating manic depression. In reviewing the medical literature on the use of lithium, which consisted of only three or four studies at the time, I learned that this alkali metal could be pharmaceutically compounded and administered to manic-depressive patients by mouth in capsule form.

Not long after, I initiated the first American psychiatric-controlled research studies of the use of lithium in patients with bipolar disorder. A few years after my initial studies, while serving as chief of research in internal medicine at Columbia Presbyterian Medical Center's department of psychiatry and the New York State Psychiatric Institute, I began to design and execute numerous long-term lithium carbonate trials in manic-depressive, unipolar, and schizophrenic patients. In the initial trials, manic-depressive patients had an immediate (3 to 10 days) and dramatic response to lithium, whereas patients with schizophrenia did not. My team and I thereafter did a 4-year study on lithium and unipolar disorder patients, and we found that there was also *mild* prevention of episodes of unipolar depression. By 1970, while I served on the American Psychiatric Association's Lithium Task Force with four American colleagues, the FDA officially approved lithium for the treatment of acute mania.

During the 1970s, it was apparent that psychiatry was going through a difficult transition and suffering from an identity crisis. While many psychiatrists, psychologists, and psychoanalysts held on to Freud's psychoanalytic explanation of the major mood disorders, there was compelling scientific evidence to the contrary. The medical model with an emphasis on heredity and brain chemistry began to replace Freud, and the age of psychopharmacology was born.

The overall impact of lithium at this point was to revolutionize diagnosis and treatment in psychiatry. In my psychiatric experience then and even today, lithium is the only medication I know of that is a specific treatment for a specific major mental illness. Lithium is also a diagnostic tool—if a person responds right away, chances are more likely that their condition is Bipolar I or II. If they don't respond, chances are it is schizophrenia. In this light, lithium revolutionized the diagnosis and treatment of two of the world's major mental illnesses in psychiatry: manic depression (bipolar disorder) and schizophrenia.

Unlike most other psychopharmacologic agents, lithium appeared to work directly on the core of the illness—though it's still a mystery as to exactly how it does so. The phenothiazines, some anticonvulsants, and the atypical antipsychotics, on the other hand, seemed to work more around the illness, suppressing it but also causing undesirable side effects such as fatigue, weight gain, or alterations in blood biochemistries.

Specificity

The idea of specificity of the lithium ion for mania has preoccupied clinical researchers over time and has been debated since Dr. Cade's original study. Dr. Cade himself believed lithium to be specific for mania, as do I to this very day. In fact, after treating and supervising the treatment of more than 8,000 patients with bipolar and unipolar disorder over many decades, I believe lithium is quite precise in treating the classic bipolar patient. It is most effective when the patient is healthy and compliant to taking the right dosage and getting blood levels of the medication checked regularly, and if there are no coexisting medical or psychiatric conditions.

While some psychiatrists prefer to use the newer mood stabilizers, as one who conducted the first studies of lithium in bipolar disorder in the United States, I still believe that lithium is the gold standard of treatment for bipolar disorder. In that light, I believe that lithium remains clearly underutilized because the older attending psychiatrists have not adequately trained young doctors as to lithium's proper use. Not only is lithium effective in reducing symptoms and frequency of episodes with a response rate of 70 to 80 percent for the initial manic phase, it effectively reduces the risk of suicide at least sixfold.[1] In that light, lithium acts both as treatment and preventative therapy. Patients who take lithium do not have the "drugged" feeling commonly reported with so many potent previously used major tranquilizers. Fortunately, the newer anticonvulsants and atypical psychotics have replaced those older tranquilizers, and their side effects are much milder and more easily tolerated by the patient. Anyone who takes lithium must remain diligent in having weekly to monthly blood levels of the drug monitored by a highly capable physician, as the medication can be toxic to persons with heart or kidney disease.

In addition, any medical condition that perturbs the electrolyte balance in the body, such as vomiting, diarrhea, or dehydration, can affect lithium balance and lead to lithium toxicity. In fact, lithium can be potentially damaging to the kidneys (where it is metabolized) and the thyroid. This is why I tell all patients who take lithium to drink 8 glasses of fluids daily and eat three normal meals, all of which will provide adequate salt and fluids for normal lithium metabolism. Because of lithium's high toxicity, blood levels need to be very carefully monitored by an experienced psychopharmacologist.

MOOD-STABILIZING MEDICATIONS

A mood-stabilizing medication works to normalize all phases of bipolar disorder, effectively treating and preventing bipolar mood states that swing back and forth between unwelcome spells of depression to the enjoyable periods of hypomania to the soaring elation that can even become psychotic. This medication also helps to improve behavior and, ultimately, social interactions. In contrast to an antidepressant, a mood-stabilizing medication may be appropriate for Bipolar II hypomanic or manic, as it does not increase the risk of cycling or switching into another mood state and does not exacerbate any phase of illness. Sometimes mood stabilizers are considered to be "augmenters," as they boost the performance of another medication, helping to keep the patient's moods stabilized. Patients with Bipolar II who suffer with depression may take a mood stabilizer to modulate mood, along with an antidepressant to lift the depressed mood.

While lithium is considered to be the only true mood stabilizer in all phases of bipolar treatment, including mania and depression, there are other commonly used mood stabilizers including Depakote (valproic acid) and Tegretol (carbamazepine). Even more recent developments among the class of mood stabilizers are the drugs Lamictal (lamotrigine) and Trileptal (oxcarbazepine). Several of the newer atypical antipsychotics (also called second-generation antipsychotics) are generally given during the agitated state of mania or depression, as well as to patients with other agitated psychotic disorders such as schizophrenia or Alzheimer's disease; these include Zyprexa (olanzapine), Seroquel (quetiapine), Geodon (ziprasidone), Risperdal (risperidone), and Abilify (aripiprazole).

Anticonvulsants

Anticonvulsants were increasingly used as mood stabilizers during the late '80s and '90s, but their current use is clearly in decline—mostly due to the high cost compared to lithium and their side effects of weight gain. While the mechanism of action is not completely understood, it is speculated that the anticonvulsants work outside the brain cell on the neurotransmitters gamma-aminobutyric acid (GABA) and glutamate. These neurotransmitters, in turn, regulate the ion channels leading into the brain cell, including calcium, sodium, chloride, and potassium.

Many doctors favor prescribing the anticonvulsant Lamictal (lamotrigine) as a mood stabilizer for their Bipolar II patients, and the drug may be as effective as or more effective than lithium in some Bipolar II patients, particularly those with rapid-cycling, although all of the data still is not in. It is thought that Lamictal has a strong antidepressant and weak antimanic effect in bipolar disorder, too.

Anticonvulsants Commonly Used as Mood Stabilizers

GENERIC NAME	TRADE NAME
Carbamazepine	Tegretol, Equetro
Divalproex sodium (valproic acid)	Depakote
Gabapentin	Neurontin*
Lamotrigine	Lamictal
Oxcarbazepine	Trileptal
Topiramate	Topamax*

*Used by some doctors but not approved by the FDA for bipolar.

Over the past 2 decades, the anticonvulsants Depakote and Tegretol have been proven effective in some patients with Bipolar I disorder if lithium, most experts' first choice, is refused or cannot be administered due to laboratory lithium testing being unavoidable; if the patient is lithium intolerant, or if the patient has a medical condition that can promote lithium toxicity. The anticonvulsants are also the first choice for patients who develop a serious rash, alopecia, or impaired kidney function while on lithium and can no longer tolerate the drug.

In a multicenter study evaluating lamotrigine monotherapy in Bipolar I disorder, Joseph R. Calabrese, MD, and his colleagues at Case Western Reserve University in Cleveland concluded that lamotrigine monotherapy is an effective treatment for bipolar depression.[2]

While Lamictal may delay the onset of mood episodes in some Bipolar II patients, it has not been found to be an effective treatment for stopping an acute manic episode. In that regard, lithium would still be my (and most experts') drug of choice for most patients with Bipolar I mania in combination with an atypical antipsychotic, then followed by Depakote and Tegretal.

Antipsychotics and Benzodiazepines

Psychiatrists have been using the typical, or conventional, antipsychotic medications such as Haldol (haloperidol) and Risperdal (risperidone), as well as the atypical, or newer, ones, including Zyprexa, Abilify, Seroquel, and Geodon, to treat the acute mania associated with Bipolar I. The benzodiazepines belong to a group of medications called central nervous system (CNS) depressants, which act on neurotransmitters to slow down normal brain function. Doctors commonly use CNS depressants to treat anxiety and sleep disorders, and they may be an effective alternative or adjunctive therapy in some Bipolar I patients with acute mania. Some commonly used benzodiazepines include Klonopin (clonazepam), Ativan (lorazepam), Xanax, and Valium. These drugs are all habit-forming/addictive and must be used only during the acute phase of the illness and not as long-term medications.

Commonly Used Typical and Atypical Antipsychotics

Typical Antipsychotics (Older Medications)

GENERIC NAME	TRADE NAME
Chlorpromazine and other phenothiazines	Thorazine
Fluphenazine	Permitil, Prolixin
Haloperidol	Haldol
Perphenazine	Trilafon
Resperidone	Respirdal
Thioridazine	Mellaril
Trifluoperazine	Stelazine

Atypical Antipsychotics
(Newer Medications)

GENERIC NAME	TRADE NAME
Aripiprazole	Abilify
Olanzapine	Zyprexa
Quetiapine fumarate	Seroquel
Ziprasidone	Geodon

Benzodiazepines Commonly Used for Anxiety
(All Potentially Addictive)

GENERIC NAME	TRADE NAME
Alprazolam	Xanax
Buspirone	BuSpar
Chlordiazepoxide-methscopolamn	Librax, Libritabs, Librium
Clonazepam	Klonopin
Diazepam	Valium
Halazepam	Paxipam
Lorazepam	Ativan
Oxazepam	Serax
Prazepam	Centrax
Propranolol	Inderal (for social anxiety)
Venlafaxine	Effexor (antidepressant also approved for anxiety)

Commonly Used Sleep Medications

Non-Habit Forming

GENERIC NAME	TRADE NAME
Mirtazapine	Remeron (atypical antidepressant)
Quetiapine fumarate	Seroquel (atypical antipsychotic)
Trazadone	Dyserel (antidepressant)

Purported to Be Non-Habit Forming

GENERIC NAME	TRADE NAME
Eszopicione	Lunesta
Zaleplon	Sonata

Habit-Forming

GENERIC NAME	TRADE NAME
Chloral hydrate	Noctec
Flurazepam HCl	Dalmane
Temazepam	Restoril
Triazolam	Halcion
Zolpidem	Ambien (mildly habit forming)

Antidepressant Medications

Many patients who come to my New York office have failed to get relief for the depressive phase of their bipolar illness, even though they have seen as many as 8 to 10 doctors. Some have taken up to 12 medications, yet none have worked satisfactorily to restore their normal mood without side effects. About 30 percent of depressed patients who take antidepressant medications do not improve at all. This may be because of the patient's particular psychological resistance or biological makeup or because the drug has too many side effects that make the patient uncomfortable. Or the patient may have a serious medical problem such as heart disease or liver or kidney disease that makes some antidepressants unsafe. Sometimes the doctor chooses the wrong antidepressant, or the right antidepressant in the wrong dosage, or does not administer the antidepressant for at least 6 weeks at the highest dose tolerable to achieve full therapeutic results.

Commonly and Uncommonly Used Antidepressants

Monoamine Oxidase Inhibitors (MAOIs)*

GENERIC NAME	TRADE NAME
Isocarboxazid	Marplan
Phenelzine	Nardil
Tranylcypromine	Parnate

Tricyclic and Quadracyclic Antidepressants**

GENERIC NAME	TRADE NAME
Amitriptyline	Elavil
Amoxapine	Asendin
Clomipramine	Anafranil
Desipramine	Norpramin
Doxepin	Adapin, Sinequan
Imipramine	Tofranil
Maprotiline	Ludiomil
Nortriptyline	Aventyl, Pamelor
Protriptyline	Vivactil
Trimipramine	Surmontil

Selective Serotonin Reuptake Inhibitors (SSRIs)***

GENERIC NAME	TRADE NAME
Citalopram hydrobromide	Celexa
Escitalopram oxalate	Lexapro
Fluoxetine	Prozac
Fluvoxamine	Luvox
Paroxetine	Paxil
Sertraline	Zoloft

Miscellaneous Antidepressants

GENERIC NAME	TRADE NAME
Bupropion	Wellbutrin, Zyban
Duloxetine[†]	Cymbalta[†]
Mirtazapine	Remeron
Trazodone	Desyrel
Venlafaxine[†]	Effexor[†]
Fluoxetine and olanzapine	Symbyax (combination)

*Rarely used today.
**Still used but less commonly used than the SSRIs.
***Starting in low doses with very careful monitoring, these antidepressants are often used in Bipolar II if a primary mood stabilizer is in place.
†Serotonin-norepinephrine reuptake inhibitor (SNRI)

Stimulants Often Used to Step Up or Boost the Antidepressant Drug Action

GENERIC NAME	TRADE NAME
Methylphenidate	Ritalin
Modafinil	Provigil

I discussed the history of antidepressants in chapter 2 and how the various types of medications work differently in the brain to affect neurotransmitters and boost mood. Yet before I give an antidepressant, I do a thorough review of the patient's personal medical and family history. If the patient has been diagnosed with bipolar disorder or has a family history of mood disorders, then I prescribe a mood stabilizer with the antidepressant, if in the depressant phase, to keep the patient's mood from extending too high (what I have labeled as Bipolar III, see page 60). I then start the antidepressant in very low doses with careful monitoring.

I explain to the patient his or her chances of recovery. I find that depressive symptoms such as weight loss, late insomnia (early morning awakening), loss of appetite, and slowed physical responses usually respond well to an antidepressant. Those patients who have many neurotic symptoms, hypochondria, hysterical traits, severe personality conflicts, or a great deal of hostility do not, in general, respond as well and often become what we call treatment resistant.

When I undertake treatment of a patient, a nurse obtains blood in our on-site laboratory and testing is done for certain medications. Initially, this is done every week, then every 2 weeks and then monthly, to continue monitoring the quantity of medication in the blood that is getting to the brain. This becomes even more important if the patient is not responding to the drug, to ensure that a therapeutic level has been reached. Blood levels tell me if the patient is taking the prescribed amount of medication, overdosing, or reaching too high a level because of his own metabolism. Older patients need to be especially monitored for maximum safety (see pages 225 to 231). Only some of the antidepressant medications can be monitored in the blood.

2004 EXPERT CONSENSUS

The Expert Consensus Guidelines give practical clinical instruction for treating the major mental disorders based on a wide survey of the best expert opinion. The 2004 Expert Consensus Guideline Series for Treatment of Bipolar Disorder, led by Paul

Keck, MD, of the University of Cincinnati, consists of survey-based expert opinions from 47 national bipolar experts. The guidelines conclude that for euphoric mania and hypomania in Bipolar I and Bipolar II disorder without a history of rapid-cycling, lithium appears to be the treatment of choice by those experts surveyed, with Depakote another first-line option. For long-term maintenance therapy after a depressive episode in Bipolar II disorder, the doctors surveyed agreed with my own personal findings in conducting scientific trials with lithium and Lamictal on bipolar patients; if lithium alone or in combination with an antidepressant fails, Lamictal monotherapy can be employed, watching carefully for allergies or signs of skin rash where the unusual occurence of Stevens-Johnson syndrome can be fatal. The reason for Lamictal is that lithium often dampens the bipolar beneficial hypomania, whereas Lamictal does not.

The expert consensus gave less support to including an atypical antipsychotic (for example, Zyprexa, Seroquel, Abilify, and Geodon) in maintenance treatment for a patient with Bipolar II disorder in great part due to the serious concern by the public and physicians of the side effects of obesity and diabetes due to these drugs. For duration of treatment after response in Bipolar II depression, experts were inclined to continue treatment with a mood stabilizer for a somewhat shorter period. If a patient without a history of rapid-cycling has severe Bipolar II depression, 40 percent of the experts questioned in this consensus said they would continue treatment with antidepressants indefinitely.[4]

I am in agreement with most of the expert consensus but favor the use of lithium as the primary maintenance treatment of Bipolar II as well as in Bipolar I. Nevertheless, I never hesitate to add either drug (Lamictal or lithium) to the opposite if there are breakthrough episodes or if I have difficulty controlling the moodswings or stabilizing the patient. In addition, I do not hesitate to add an atypical antipsychotic in small dosages. In highly creative Bipolar IIB types, I favor using small doses of lithium or

Lamictal. If the patient insists on taking no medication, I often agree but only if he or she agrees to be monitored by me periodically and to see a psychologist. It is not unusual for patients with Bipolar IIB to maximize their creativity when they are taking no medications whatsoever.

Since all of the mood stabilizers appear to be equally effective, the choice is often made based upon previous history and response, family history and response to a given antidepressant, side-effect profiles, and coexisting medical illnesses.

The Hope of Clinical Trials

After struggling for years to find medications that are highly effective yet without side effects, many patients volunteer to participate in clinical trials in the hopes of finding an undiscovered drug that will resolve their mood disorder. It is well known that about 20 to 30 percent of all depressed patients who take antidepressant medication do not improve from it. This may be because of the person's particular psychological resistance or biological makeup, or because the drug has too many side effects that make the patient uncomfortable and are not acceptable. Or the patient may have a medical problem such as heart, liver, or kidney disease that makes some antidepressants unsafe.

Evaluating Investigational Drugs

Major pharmaceutical companies constantly develop new medications, which must be proven safe and effective for human use before doctors are permitted to write prescriptions for them. Through clinical trials, under carefully controlled conditions, researchers can evaluate new investigational drugs under development. Such study drugs offer a no-cost alternative and are accompanied by free medical and psychiatric evaluations as part of the clinical trials.

A clinical trial is a carefully designed study that tests the effects of a medication, medical treatment, or device on a group of volunteers. Clinical trials measure the ability of a drug, treatment, or device to treat a condition, its safety, and its possible side effects. Most trials involve new medications not available to the public. (These are phases I to III trials.) Other studies focus on existing marketed medications (phase IV), which are being evaluated for their effectiveness compared to other medications and also for new indications. When a patient is not responding well to traditional antidepressants or other medications, I sometimes suggest that he or she participate in a clinical trial study of a still unmarketed drug conducted by my own research group.

There are always new antidepressant, antianxiety, and antibipolar compounds under development. Many are being developed in my research offices, Fieve Clinical Services, which are adjacent to but separate from my private practice on the Upper East Side of Manhattan. It is the hope of researchers that these new compounds will be more rapid in onset, prove more effective than their predecessors, and have fewer side effects than ones currently in use. To the observer, bipolar disorder and major depression have a lot in common. However, we believe that different brain hormones and biochemical mechanisms are responsible for different depressive conditions, so new drugs are constantly being developed to target these. Many of the new drugs under investigation are still without a name and bear research numbers from pharmaceutical laboratories. Most of the drugs being investigated in phases I through IV have already been taken by several thousand volunteers and patients in the United States or worldwide after having been first tested in animal studies at the pharmaceutical company.

I specialize in the treatment of many so-called treatment-refractory mood disorders. For these patients with "hopeless" bipolar disorder and depression, participation in a clinical trial is like coming to a "court of last resort." We are always optimistic that some of the newest medications undergoing clinical investigation will work faster than the older, traditional medications, finally giving these patients relief from their moodswings.

Some of the FDA-Approved Drugs for Treatment of Bipolar Mania and Depression

1970: Lithium approved for the treatment of mania in bipolar disorder.

1995: Depakote* (divalproex sodium) approved for the treatment of the manic episodes of bipolar disorder.

2000: Zyprexa* (olanzapine) approved as a monotherapy for the short-term treatment of acute manic episodes associated with bipolar disorder.

2003: Lamictal (lamotrigine) approved for the long-term maintenance of Bipolar I disorder.

2003: Zyprexa* (olanzapine) approved for use in combination with lithium or valproate for the treatment of acute manic episodes with Bipolar I disorder.

2003: Symbyax* (Prozac and Zyprexa combination) approved to treat the depressive phase of bipolar disorder.

2003: Risperdal (risperidone) approved for monotherapy (alone) or in combination with lithium or valproate for the short-term treatment of acute mania or mixed episodes with Bipolar I disorder, also known as bipolar mania.

Sometimes, within even a few days, rather than weeks, treatment-refractory patients enrolled in clinical trials may begin to feel better on the trial medication. They may feel a surge of energy, a lifting of mood, less anxiety, better sleep, and more balanced mood for the first time in months or years. In our clinical trials, the improvement in symptoms and side effects is documented and rated with measuring scales given by trained raters. We then give this data to the pharmaceutical company for analysis.

2004: Seroquel* (quetiapine) approved for monotherapy of mania associated with bipolar disorder but not for treatment of bipolar depression.

2004: Geodon* (ziprasidone HCl) approved by the FDA to treat bipolar mania, including manic and mixed episodes.

2004: Abilify* (aripiprazole) approved for treatment of acute bipolar mania, including manic and mixed episodes associated with bipolar disorder.

2004: Zyprexa* (olanzapine) approved for acute agitation in patients suffering with bipolar disorder; oral Zyprexa is approved for long-term therapy.

2004: Equetro (extended-release carbamazepine capsules) approved for the treatment of acute manic and mixed episodes associated with Bipolar I disorder.

2005: Abilify* (aripiprazole) approved with an expanded indication allowing its use for maintaining efficacy in patients with Bipolar I disorder who had been stabilized and maintained after a recent manic or mixed episode for at least 6 weeks.

*Under investigation by the FDA due to serious side effects of obesity and diabetes in some patients

As a board-certified psychiatrist, trained in psychopharmacology and internal medicine, I am the principal investigator of Fieve Clinical Services and oversee many trials being conducted simultaneously at our research site. Other investigators at our clinical research center often include board-certified psychiatrists (including a pediatric/adolescent psychiatrist), internists, and neurologists who have training from or are affiliated with top New York hospitals such as Columbia Presbyterian, New York Cornell, Mount Sinai, Bellevue/NYU Medical Center,

St. Vincent's Hospital, and Gracie Square Hospital. There are many clinics across the nation that specialize in drug research. Talk to your primary care physician to see if there is one in your area.

Stages of Testing

Within any drug-development process, there are specific stages through which the drug must pass. At each critical stage, a certain threshold must be attained before the process can advance to the next level. Before Phase I clinical testing in humans, medications are tested in laboratory animals. Phase I clinical studies follow and are commonly referred to as the "first in man" studies. During Phase I, 40 to 100 healthy volunteers are given test doses of the drug for the first time in humans in a controlled inpatient hospital setting to determine safety, metabolization, duration of action, rate of excretion, or possible side effects. In Phase II, the drug is given to a small group of hospital inpatients who are actually suffering from the condition the drug is intended to treat. Later on, the Phase II drug is used with outpatients.

Phase III is the final stage of testing prior to the FDA application for approval submitted by the pharmaceutical company. At this stage, data are accumulated on hundreds or even thousands of patient volunteers, with the condition being investigated in 10 to 50 sites across the United States. During this phase, patient recruitment requires close attention to diagnosis and inclusion-exclusion detail. At the completion of this phase, the drug sponsor will assemble all of the relevant data from the pre-clinical and clinical trial process and submit a New Drug Application to the FDA. Once approval is obtained, the FDA requires pharmaceutical companies to conduct limited post-marketing, or Phase IV, studies, primarily to determine if there are any safety issues that arise from long-term use or interactions with other drugs taken by patients in the real world.

Clinical trials are typically sponsored by the pharmaceutical companies, but federal agencies such as the FDA, universities, hospitals, and medical foundations may also sponsor trials and submit the protocol first to the FDA for approval to proceed.

People with the condition being studied as well as healthy volunteers can participate in a clinical trial. The FDA has very strict requirements that specify which studies involve healthy volunteers and which studies involve patients with specific medical and psychiatric conditions.

Each study has specific requirements for participants, such as age, gender, and medical/psychiatric condition. Initially, a research assistant will ask basic information about your current condition and medications during a brief interview by phone or in person that will allow him or her to decide whether you are a good candidate to participate in the trial. If you qualify based on the phone screen, you will be scheduled for an appointment to speak to the research psychiatrist or the principal investigator for a diagnostic evaluation and a determination as to whether you qualify to participate in the trial. During the appointment with the research psychiatrist, the study will be explained to you in detail and you will be given the opportunity to decide if you want to participate in it.

My research team at Fieve Clinical Services is trained in medical and psychiatric conditions and the technical aspects of the protocols we are investigating. The team explains to all participants everything about the trial, discusses what to expect, and answers any questions or concerns the participants might have. When you make the appointment, they will tell you what to expect in the first visit.

Added Patient Benefit

Perhaps the greatest benefit of participating in a clinical trial is having the opportunity to receive cutting-edge psychiatric medicine for treatment of your condition at no cost. In some Phase IV trials, the FDA has already approved the medication for other nonpsychiatric uses in the United States, and the trial now being conducted is to determine the effectiveness of the drug in treating mood disorders or anxiety. Many effective drugs that are approved by the FDA for one symptom or illness are often found to be useful in treating other problems or illnesses. For instance, the antidepressant Wellbutrin is used to treat depression and also to help cigarette smokers kick the habit. Anticonvulsants, originally approved for seizure disorders, are highly effective in modulating mood in bipolar disorder. In addition, in most cases, once the trial is completed, which takes 8 weeks, you will have the opportunity to keep receiving the medication being studied at no cost for a period of time, along with several sessions with a psychiatrist at no cost. Later low-cost follow-up treatment is also offered.

The government has strict guidelines and safeguards to protect people who choose to participate in clinical trials. Every clinical trial in the United States must be approved and monitored by an Institutional Review Board (IRB) to make sure the risks are as low as possible and are worth the potential benefits. An IRB is an independent committee of physicians, statisticians, community advocates, and others that ensures that a clinical trial is ethical and protects the rights of study participants. All institutions that conduct or support biomedical research involving people must, by federal regulation, have an IRB that initially approves and periodically reviews the research.

All information collected during your participation in the trial is held confidentially. (A unique code is assigned to you that will be used on all information related to your care.) At any point in time, if you so desire, you can withdraw from the study. That is your right.

If you are considering joining a clinical trial, the research staff will give you informed consent documents that include the details about all aspects of the study. Since joining a clinical trial is an important decision, you should ask the research team any questions you may have about the study and the consent forms before you make a decision. You may refer to my Web site at www.FieveClinical.com or check page 254, which list other Web sites that will allow you to get access to clinical trials in your own state.

For Those with Bipolar II and Their Family Members

- Bipolar II does not go away nor is there a cure. It is a chronic, lifelong problem that needs a proper diagnosis and long-term medical management and treatment. If you are taking a prescribed medication, it is necessary to take this drug daily, even when your mood is normal and you feel well, to avoid future moodswings.

- If you still have symptoms that are not improving even with medication, talk openly with your doctor about changing the medication or trying a combination of medications. Many times it takes several tries to find the most effective mood medication that gives the greatest benefit with the fewest side effects. Be your own advocate and talk with your doctor until you feel your best.

- If you are not responding to the prescribed medications, ask your doctor about the availability of clinical trials for Bipolar II disorder in your area and enlist in one of these. Oftentimes, the new medications used in clinical trials can help patients who are difficult to treat. Every time a new drug is investigated and then developed, hundreds of thousands of Bipolar II patients may be successfully helped. When your medication is effective, it allows you to work more efficiently and have stronger relationships. You can become hopeful about the future—a future *without* out-of-control moods.

- If you are not seeing a mood specialist, ask your primary care physician for a referral to a psychopharmacologist. Working with this expert, you can find the right mood stabilizer or combination of medications that have the lowest incidences of side effects. In my years of practice, I have found that patients are far more likely to stay compliant to their medication regimens when there are few side effects.

CHAPTER 9

SPECIAL SITUATIONS THAT COMPLICATE A BIPOLAR DIAGNOSIS

Detection of bipolar disorder is the first step in preventing further mood episodes. But treating bipolar signs and symptoms presents a unique challenge under certain circumstances. In this chapter, I will discuss these special situations that must be handled differently. After reading this chapter, I urge you to write down your personal concerns and questions about treatment and then share these with your doctor.

PREGNANCY AND BIPOLAR II

When Bipolar II disorder is properly diagnosed, it is a highly treatable condition. Yet there are some special circumstances when Bipolar II is especially difficult to manage. For instance, the median age of onset for bipolar disorder is 25[1]—around the time when some women of childbearing age might begin to consider marriage and starting families. While bipolar medications keep the patient's mood stabilized, they can greatly increase the risk of fetal malformations if taken during pregnancy. Women with Bipolar II must know the facts about these medications and learn how to work with their doctors in weighing the risks and benefits to mother and baby.

When I initially diagnose a woman of childbearing age with Bipolar II, I require her to participate in ongoing counseling with my staff psychologist to discuss her sexual health. Through this extensive counseling, they discuss birth control and sexually transmitted diseases, the risk of having a child with bipolar disorder should the patient get pregnant, and the need to come off mood-stabilizing drugs before making the decision to conceive. The psychologist and I work closely with the patient to ensure that she has optimum control of her bipolar moodswings and is also well educated about the illness and how treatment can influence contraception and family planning.

Contraception

Not only is Bipolar II more common in women than in men, but women often present with different clinical features, perhaps because of hormonal treatments and reproductive events. For example, women are more likely to experience rapid-cycling and antidepressant-induced mania, and they respond differently to treatment.

Additionally, several bipolar medications such as Topamax, Tegretol, and Trileptal can increase the metabolism of oral contraceptives, rendering the birth control ineffective. Women who take these medications for their bipolar disorder cannot rely on oral contraceptives to prevent a pregnancy. In addition, oral contraceptives can slow down the elimination of benzodiazepines from the body, which can lead to impairment of the woman's cognitive and psychomotor abilities. There are safe options for contraception, but these depend on the woman's diagnosis and the specific medications she takes. Working closely with an ob-gyn and psychopharmacologist, almost all women can find safe and effective methods of birth control while remaining compliant to the necessary mood medications.

Genetic Counseling

Because of the strong genetic loading of bipolar disorder, it is important that couples have a complete understanding of the genetics of this mood disorder, which I discussed in chapter 3. Before getting pregnant, all of my Bipolar II patients are urged to make an appointment with a genetic counselor at Columbia Presbyterian Medical Center. This health professional has specialized training in the area of medical genetics and counseling and helps to identify families at risk for inherited conditions such as bipolar disorder.

The counseling sessions are especially important when the bipolar patient has a spouse with a family history of bipolar disorder and/or depression. After studying both family histories, the genetic counselor will explain the probability of a child having bipolar disorder, depression, or any of the other conditions that are common in bipolar families. This knowledge helps parents watch for signs and symptoms as the child develops so they can seek medical treatment early in the illness when treatment is most effective in managing or even stopping the mood symptoms.

Mood-Stabilizing Drugs and Pregnancy

Twenty-nine-year-old Jessica has Bipolar II and had been stabilized on the anticonvulsant Depakote for 3 years. As I noted in chapter 8, physicians and psychiatrists often use anticonvulsants when a patient can't tolerate lithium.

Jessica had been given Depakote because she had experienced two episodes of hypomania and a lengthy period of moderate depression that had resulted in a 2-week hospitalization when she was in college. When she became my patient, she decided she wanted to remain on Depakote, which seemed to be working well. After she got married, Jessica and her husband talked to me about pregnancy. I told them that I strongly recommend that patients not get pregnant while taking any bipolar medication. Depakote may cause birth defects in some babies.

Unfortunately, after being married just 6 months, Jessica unexpectedly became pregnant. Because she was still on the Depakote, she was very upset that she might have a baby with cardiovascular problems or other malformations.

I discussed the options for the pregnancy with Jessica and her husband. They decided that Jessica would go off Depakote during the pregnancy to make sure the baby was healthy. I discussed with them the moodswings Jessica most likely would encounter while off medication. I also recommended that they come to my office for counseling every other week throughout the pregnancy to monitor her moodswings off medication. Her husband volunteered to come for counseling with her, as he assumed that he might be able to identify and deal with the moodswings she was having and could help Jessica to cope with them in this way.

During the pregnancy, Jessica did experience some uncontrollable moodswings, but nothing that we could not handle as a "team." For instance, she had several weeks of feeling very low and exhausted in the first trimester. But this is a time when even women of normal mood might feel fatigued and moody because of the dramatic changes in hormones. She had one period of very high energy in her middle trimester where it was difficult for her to sleep for about a week. Jessica said that she used that time to plan the baby's nursery and did yoga postures to try to relax at night. With her husband's help, Jessica made it through to the delivery without medication, and they were thrilled when they had a very healthy baby girl. Unlike many women today, Jessica did not breastfeed, a choice she and her husband made several months before the birth, so that she could immediately go back on Depakote. I commended Jessica and her husband for making very responsible decisions. They did all in their power to make sure that the baby was healthy ensuring a healthy postpartum period for both mother and newborn.

Ideally, all bipolar patients should stop all medications before they conceive. I instruct my patients to slowly taper off the bipolar medications in preparation for pregnancy and to allow a period of time for detoxification to clear the body of the medication. Stopping medications abruptly can lead to a greater risk of a mood episode occurring. Once a patient is off all bipolar medication and then conceives, I work closely with the pregnant woman, her ob-gyn, and the family to ensure a safe and healthy pregnancy, delivery, and postpartum period.

So often, the added stress of pregnancy can affect the bipolar patient when mood-stabilizing medications must be discontinued for this period of time. Pregnant bipolar patients sometimes turn to illegal drugs or alcohol as a way of escaping from the hypomania or depression—but both of these substances increase the risk of birth defects and can exacerbate the high or low mood. Education before pregnancy is crucial to avoid a mental health crisis.

If the patient gets pregnant unexpectedly while on medication, as Jessica did, then she must consider the effects of the specific drug on the unborn fetus; the most common problem is cardiovascular malformation. She can then weigh her options of whether she wants to continue the pregnancy. I wish there was a sure and positive outcome for these patients and their pregnancies, but the latest scientific findings give *no* safety guarantees when it comes to taking the medications during pregnancy. I have heard anecdotal reports of patients taking medication after the first trimester with no harm to the fetus. But, again, there is no assurance that the fetus will be safe from birth defects.

Though I strongly advise against it, if a woman does choose to stay on lithium, I recommend that she have a few tests: a maternal serum a-fetoprotein screening for neural tube defects before the 20th week of gestation with amniocentesis and targeted sonogram for elevated a-fetoprotein values. Another important test to detect cardiac abnormalities in the fetus, no matter which drug the expectant mother is taking, is the high-resolution ultrasound examination at 16 to 18 weeks. In addition, it is important that the patient have regular monitoring of the maternal serum levels and that medication dosages are adjusted if needed. At delivery, the mother's body fluid rapidly shifts, which can greatly increase lithium levels. A psychopharmacologist should be at the delivery to manage the dosage and ensure hydration.

The stress of labor and delivery, along with the first weeks of the postpartum period, are apt to increase the likelihood of escalating moodswings, particularly if the mother is unable to get the necessary sleep. The postpartum period is often linked to mild but swift moodswings from sadness to elation, irritability, crying, and insomnia. In fact, 40 to 80 percent of all normal women develop mild changes within 2 to 3 days after delivery. Symptoms usually peak on the 5th postpartum day and resolve within 2 weeks.[2] But women with bipolar disorder have a higher rate of postpartum depression and may have a more severe form of this illness—called postpartum psychosis—which affects about one in 1,000 women with symptoms of paranoia, depressed or manic mood shifts, and/or hallucinations or delusions.

During the postpartum period, I stay particularly close to my patient, who has been well educated before pregnancy about the link between sleep habits and mood episodes. If there is a problem with mood after delivery, the patient, the family, and I must weigh the immediate benefits and risks of taking medication to modulate mood and breastfeeding the newborn. The greatest concern during breastfeeding is with lithium use, as lithium is excreted in breast milk. Still, there are no guarantees on any of the commonly used medications, as all bipolar medications are secreted in breast milk in varying degrees. When the breastfeeding mother takes bipolar medications, the infant has the potential for getting the pharmacological effects, a life-threatening rash, and/or other very serious symptoms. If a patient must take medication, then she should formula-feed the newborn so as to avoid risk to the child.

While there are no empirically based treatment guidelines for the management of Bipolar II during pregnancy, I tell my bipolar patients that they are likely to feel quite well throughout the pregnancy without medication. Still, I insist that they continue their frequent visits to my office for medical checkups and ongoing psychological counseling. I also ask that they communicate frequently with telephone consults, so I can monitor their daily mood and sleep habits; if patients have even subtle changes in mood and behavior, I instruct them to call me immediately. Likewise, I urge family members to report to me any noticeable signs of moodswings that a patient may not notice.

If you or a loved one is considering having a baby and Bipolar II disorder is an obstacle, talk to a bipolar expert (psychiatrist or psychopharmacologist) about your situation. While Bipolar II is a challenging mood disorder, it can become even more so during pregnancy. But if you enter into the pregnancy with knowledge and the ongoing support of your doctors and family, this situation can be passed through safely and successfully, bringing a lifetime of joy into the world for those involved.

CHILDREN, ADOLESCENTS, AND BIPOLAR II

Doctors continue to misdiagnose children and teenagers with attention-deficit/hyperactivity disorder (ADHD) or attention deficit disorder (ADD), which has symptoms similar to bipolar disorder, and improperly treat them with central nervous system stimulants such as Ritalin (methylphenidate). We now believe that many of these young people may actually have Bipolar II disorder instead of ADD or ADHD. The incorrectly used stimulants can increase their anger, out-of-control behavior, and even thoughts of suicide.

As I discussed in chapter 2, depression comes in three forms—major depressive disorder, dysthymic disorder (mild, chronic depression), and bipolar depressive disorder. While we are learning more about Bipolar II in children and teens, it is still extremely difficult to diagnose this ailment in young people, especially when moodiness and acting out against authority are two traits that coexist with most normal adolescents. It is hard to tell if the preteen or teenager is going through a difficult but normal developmental phase or is suffering from actual bipolar depression.

From the age of 2, Brienna was conspicuously overactive. Her parents became exhausted trying to keep up with her, and it seemed that the only time she was still was during sleep. Brienna was highly irritable, lashing out at family and friends, and she had a tough time in preschool and kindergarten, where teachers often gave her time out for screaming or hitting other children. Twice administrators asked Brienna to leave a private school where she was enrolled. By the time she started first grade, she had already seen a number of child psychologists. Exasperated by her behavior, her first-grade teacher suggested that Brienna be put on Ritalin, an addictive stimulant commonly used for attention-deficit/hyperactivity disorder. ADHD often mimics bipolar disorder with rapid speech, physical restlessness, extreme energy, trouble focusing, irritability, and sometimes defiant behavior. But bipolar disorder is primarily a mood disorder, whereas ADHD mostly affects attention and behavior. While ADHD is chronic, bipolar disorder is usually episodic with periods of normal mood interspersed with the depression or hypomania.

Many times, teachers will tell parents during a conference that they suspect ADHD in a student. The parents then rush to the pediatrician upon the teacher's "diagnosis" and return with a large supply of Ritalin or other stimulant medication. A nonmedical member of the teaching staff then gives the child the stimulant each day, and no one is aware that the powerful medication may exacerbate symptoms of childhood bipolar disorder. This can result in the Bipolar II child becoming extremely active, volatile, angry, and out of control.

It is widely known (and accepted) that schoolteachers and psychologists are prone to recommending Ritalin and similar medications for any child or adolescent exhibiting restlessness, trouble focusing, or hyperactivity. Ritalin does have benefits when used correctly, as it increases mental alertness and helps some children function better in school. However, while we see the aforementioned symptoms in ADHD, we also see them in early Bipolar II disorder. That is why a thorough diagnostic evaluation and, in particular, a family history by a psychopharmacologist are necessary before giving a child any medication for these symptoms.

After Brienna and her parents began the complicated schedule of medications, the child went from being sluggish and fatigued to even more hyperactive, so they increased her dosages, as the pediatrician's nurse had instructed over the telephone. Brienna failed to learn much in school, and the school guidance counselor and psychologist both agreed that she had a serious case of ADHD.

By the time she was 9, Brienna was taking three medications: the Ritalin to treat the ADHD and remain alert during the daytime hours, a sleeping pill at night, and an antidepressant to boost her depressed mood. At this time, her parents divorced, in great part due to the stress of caring for a misdiagnosed bipolar child. She then lived part-time with one parent and part-time with the other. The complex schedule was blamed for adding to her hyperactive behavior.

By the age of 10, Brienna was hospitalized for depression, and she remained in counseling after she was released. Her doctor adjusted her medications and changed the antidepressant. A year later, Brienna reported that she felt suicidal, and she was readmitted to the hospital, but this time on a suicide watch. After she was released on large doses of the antipsychotic drug Seroquel (used to treat acute mania) and an antidepressant she did not like, she promptly refused to take any medications. That's when her parents brought her to my office for the first time, at age 11, in a mildly depressed state.

After evaluating Brienna and reviewing her medical charts, I told the young girl and her parents that I thought she might be suffering from early-onset Bipolar II disorder instead of ADHD. I noted that in her large family, there was a strong history of sociopathy, depression, and alcohol addiction, all distinct markers in bipolar families. I started Brienna on Depakote, an anticonvulsant, which made her feel fatigued in the morning and caused her to gain weight. When she refused to take the drug any longer, I switched her to lithium and Wellbutrin (an antidepressant). I saw her at four succeeding weekly visits, until her lithium blood level reached a therapeutic steady state. During the period of lithium stabilization, I also increased her dose of Wellbutrin. While starting her on these new medications, we still feared that the suicidal thoughts might return. Thus, the family, my associate psychologist, and I got Brienna to sign a contract that she would not harm herself, and she agreed to call me on my cellular any time night or day if she had suicidal thoughts.

Brienna showed mild improvement after 1 week, which developed into marked improvement by week 3 with minor complaints of side effects. In this preteen's case, the stimulant medications used to treat hyperactivity may actually have precipitated the disturbing hypomanic periods followed by depressive episodes. These obvious signs of Bipolar II had gone unnoticed because of the previously common assumption even among psychiatrists that bipolar illness appears only in late adolescence and the early to mid-twenties.

(continued on page 218)

Diagnostic Criteria for
Attention-Deficit/Hyperactivity Disorder

The following diagnostic criteria from the *DSM-IV* are used by health care professionals to make the diagnosis of ADD or ADHD. Review the specific criteria from A through E, and then talk to your child's doctor if your child has signs or symptoms of ADD or ADHD that concern you.

A. "Either 1 or 2

   1) For a diagnosis of ADD with inattention, six (or more) of the following symptoms of **inattention** have persisted for at least 6 months to a degree that is maladaptive and inconsistent with developmental level:

      a) Often fails to give close attention to details or makes careless mistakes in schoolwork, work, or other activities

      b) Often has difficulty sustaining attention in tasks or play activities

      c) Often does not seem to listen when spoken to directly

      d) Often does not follow through on instructions and fails to finish schoolwork, chores, or duties in the workplace (not due to oppositional behavior or failure to understand instructions)

      e) Often has difficulty organizing tasks and activities

      f) Often avoids, dislikes, or is reluctant to engage in tasks that require sustained mental effort (such as schoolwork or homework)

      g) Often loses things necessary for tasks or activities (e.g., toys, school assignments, pencils, books, or tools)

      h) Is often easily distracted by extraneous stimuli

      i) Is often forgetful in daily activities

   2) For the diagnosis of ADHD type with hyperactivity, six (or more) of the following symptoms of **hyperactivity-impulsivity** have persisted for at least 6 months to a degree that is maladaptive and inconsistent with developmental level:

Hyperactivity

a) Often fidgets with hands or feet or squirms in seat

b) Often leaves seat in classroom or in other situations in which remaining seated is expected

c) Often runs about or climbs excessively in situations in which it is inappropriate (in adolescents or adults, may be limited to subjective feelings of restlessness)

d) Often has difficulty playing or engaging in leisure activities quietly

e) Is often "on the go" or often acts as if "driven by a motor"

f) Often talks excessively

Impulsivity

g) Often blurts out answers before questions have been completed

h) Often has difficulty awaiting turn

i) Often interrupts or intrudes on others (e.g., butts into conversations or games)

B. Some hyperactive-impulsive or inattentive symptoms that caused impairment were present before 7 years of age.

C. Some impairment from the symptoms is present in two or more settings (e.g., at school [or work] or at home).

D. There must be clear evidence of clinically significant impairment in social, academic, or occupational functioning.

E. The symptoms do not occur exclusively during the course of a pervasive developmental disorder, schizophrenia, or other psychotic disorder and are not better accounted for by another mental disorder (e.g., mood disorder, anxiety disorder, dissociative disorder, or personality disorder)."[3]

Brienna's mood successfully stabilized on lithium and the antidepressant partly because of the excellent support of her mother and father; they were careful to insist on her keeping her appointments with me. I explained to them how to be aware of any lithium side effects. Because lithium's balance in the child's blood must be monitored carefully, I told them to call me for a medication adjustment if they were vacationing in a hot climate or if Brienna was engaged in extreme athletic activity during the summer; when sodium and fluid are lost from the body through perspiration or dehydration, the body excretes less lithium, resulting in increased serum lithium levels and the risk of lithium toxicity. When the lithium level was stabilized, Brienna came to my office for brief visits each month to check her blood lithium levels. Her mood and behavior returned to normal, and she is now doing well in school and with peer relationships.

Will Brienna continue to need this medication for her Bipolar II disorder? My guess would be yes. However, I will continue to evaluate her biochemical-behavioral status and medications periodically as she proceeds through adolescence and into young adulthood. In Brienna's case, the accompanying psychotherapy for both the patient and the family played a most important role in her compliance to medication. So often, many adolescents refuse to return to the doctor or take the much-needed prescribed medication, whereby the illness most often recurs.

Bipolar II disorder in children often is confused with other *DSM-IV* diagnoses such as ADHD, ADD, substance-induced mood disorder, oppositional defiant disorder, and conduct disorder. It is not uncommon for some of these disorders to be comorbid, or to coexist, with pediatric Bipolar II disorder.

In recent years, psychiatrists have been confronted with the problem of distinguishing between Bipolar II disorder and ADHD or ADD in children and early adolescents, as the symptoms often overlap. Sometimes the two disorders coexist, in which case individual treatments for both disorders must be used simultaneously. Like bipolar disorder, both ADHD and ADD involve symptoms such as distractibility, irritability, poor concentration, and insomnia; ADHD also has hyperactivity and impulsivity. With both ADHD and ADD, learning is difficult and grades in school begin to fall. Traditionally, ADHD and ADD are treated with amphetamine-like drugs such as Ritalin, Dexedrine and Adderall (dextroamphetamine), Strattera (atomoxetine), Concerta (methylphenidate), and Cylert (pemoline) and Provigil (modafinil), which, in my opinion, are often overused and abused when a pediatric psychopharmacologist has not made the diagnosis and treatment recommendation.

In my clinical experience, a number of these children and adolescents are not suffering from attention deficit problems at all but from the early stages of Bipolar II hypomania. Genetics play a key role in ADD, ADHD, and bipolar disorder, and a family history of bipolar illness favors a diagnosis of Bipolar II disorder. Sometimes a doctor is justified in giving a brief trial of Ritalin and, if ineffective, a separate, brief trial of lithium. If only a partial response occurs with these drugs, a combination of the two is often very effective.

Mixed Signs and Symptoms

Bipolar II is a relentless and complex illness that can happen in childhood and adolescence and completely disrupt the life of a family. Increased rates of suicide attempts and completions, poorer academic performances, disturbed interpersonal relationships, increased rates of substance abuse, and multiple hospitalizations are not uncommon if the bipolar disorder is undetected, misdiagnosed, or poorly treated.

It is difficult to diagnose children or teens with Bipolar II because the signs and symptoms may coexist with a host of other psychiatric problems, including anxiety disorders, conduct disorder, attention-deficit/hyperactivity disorder, oppositional defiant disorder, and others listed in the *DSM-IV* for children. For instance, as teens assess their future possibilities, whether starting high school, going to college, or applying for a job, they often suffer with anxiety, an uneasy feeling of worry, apprehension, and distress, often about the future. In this life transition, anxiety would be a normal feeling, one that usually resolves on its own. Anxiety, with its finger-drumming restlessness, is different from depression, with its symptoms of hopelessness, discouragement, sadness, and despair. This is why we psychiatrists classify the anxiety disorders separately from the depressive disorders.

In a primary anxiety disorder, anxiety is the primary—and often the first—symptom to appear; even though secondary depression may be present and closer to the surface, anxiety may be more obvious to the parent. Anxiety disorders, discussed on page 28, include:

- Generalized anxiety disorder (GAD)
- Phobic disorder
- Panic disorder
- Obsessive-compulsive disorder (OCD)
- Post-traumatic stress disorder (PTSD)
- Social anxiety

In children and teens, anxiety may also be one of the symptoms of a depressive disorder, but the depressed mood usually appears first as the primary symptom and is the most important part of the illness.

Teenage rebellion often mimics Bipolar II symptoms, yet it usually is not related to any major mental illness. Drug or alcohol abuse can likewise lead to symptoms that mimic Bipolar II disorder, yet it is a separate diagnostic-treatment problem altogether.

A hypomanic teen can be the extroverted leader at school as he uses charm, charisma, and passion to win students and teachers to his cause. This teen may be overly involved in clubs and sports activities, filling every time slot with another extracurricular commitment while also getting superb grades, working part-time, and volunteering on weekends for local agencies. Alternatively, the hypomanic teen may be the irritable rebel who defies authority and sneaks out of her bedroom window at night to carouse, use alcohol or recreational drugs to get high, and engage in sexual encounters. Parents must be acutely aware of such changes and the child's behaviors both at home and at school and intervene immediately should they notice a change in behavior or suspect the beginning signs of a behavioral problem or a psychiatric illness.

The depressed child or adolescent may have many physical complaints, from muscle aches, stomachaches, or headaches to being exhausted for no reason, resulting in absences from school or poor performance in school. Commonly seen are symptoms such as irritability, unexplained crying, social isolation, withdrawn and sullen behavior, and extreme sensitivity to rejection or failure, which can really describe many normal children or adolescents at various times.

Detecting Bipolar II disorder early is crucial to prevent major episodes from robbing your child of quality of life. Unlike many adults with Bipolar II disorder, whose episodes tend to be more clearly defined, children and teens with the illness often experience rapid moodswings (called rapid-cycling, see page 28) that move between depression and hypomania more than four times a year.

According to the National Institute of Mental Health, if your child or teenager has five or more of the following symptoms over a period of 2 weeks, it is important that you seek professional help.[4] With medications and/or psychotherapy, mental health professionals can help stabilize your child's moods and stop the depressed or hypomanic thoughts and behaviors.

When a child is depressed:

- He feels sad or cries a lot and his sadness doesn't go away.
- She feels guilty for no reason; she loses her confidence.
- He may complain of pain, headache, or stomachache for which no medical explanation is found.
- Life seems meaningless or like nothing good is ever going to happen again. She has a negative attitude a lot of the time, or it seems like she has no feelings.
- He doesn't feel like doing a lot of the things he used to enjoy.
- She wants to be left alone most of the time.
- He has difficulty making decisions.
- She is forgetful and cannot concentrate at school.
- He is irritable and overreacts when things don't go his way.
- Her sleep pattern changes (she sleeps a lot more or has difficulty falling asleep).
- His eating habits change (either loss of appetite or eating a lot more).
- She feels restless and tired.
- He thinks about death or feels like he is dying.
- She has thoughts about committing suicide.

When a child is hypomanic:

- He feels high as a kite . . . like he is "on top of the world."
- She has grandiose ideas about the great things she can do . . . things that she really can't do.
- He has racing thoughts and jumps from one subject to another; he talks fast and a lot.
- She is extremely social.
- He takes risks and exhibits daredevil behavior.
- She spends more money than she should from her allowance or part-time job and may be hypersexual.
- He needs little sleep because he is so "high."
- She is rebellious or irritable and can't get along with parents or teachers.
- He gets into fights with his friends or teachers.[5]

Suicidal Tendencies

Each year in the United States, approximately 2 million adolescents attempt suicide, and almost 700,000 receive medical attention for their attempt.[6] Studies show that as many as 50 percent of adolescents with bipolar disorder attempt suicide at least once.[7] In fact, bipolar disorder is the third leading cause of death among people ages 15 to 24 years. While we used to think that suicide in adolescents resulted from a stressful event such as not making the team, a romantic breakup, or failing a class, now we know that underlying psychiatric illness is the number one risk factor for adolescent suicide. In fact, psychiatric disorders such as Bipolar I and II, major depression, dysthymic disorder, or schizophrenia can be diagnosed in more than 90 percent of young people who attempt or complete suicide.

Depressed people of all ages—not just teenagers—are often suicidal; it is a key symptom of the disease. The statistics are relatively high of individuals of all ages with untreated Bipolar II disorder who attempt suicide, sometimes successfully. Some studies show that the neurotransmitter serotonin plays a central role in the neurobiology of suicide. Researchers have found lower levels of serotonin in the brain stem and cerebrospinal fluid of suicidal individuals.[8]

If your child talks about suicide, makes a suicidal gesture, or attempts suicide, take it as a serious emergency and seek immediate help from a pediatric psychiatrist/psychopharmacologist. Even if you're in doubt as to the seriousness, any talk of suicide is always an emergency. Have your child talk with a board-certified pediatric psychiatrist/psychopharmacologist immediately.

Diagnosis and Treatment

Making any kind of psychiatric diagnosis, including Bipolar II, in young children or teens is most difficult because of the normal moodswings, rebellious behavior, sulking, and alcohol and drug abuse that often occur in these early years. As always, the family history is critical in making an accurate diagnosis. I have seen many teens who were first diagnosed as schizophrenic. Upon finding out that a parent or near relative was depressed, bipolar, or an alcohol or substance abuser, I would consider whether the diagnosis wasn't really Bipolar I or II disorder. I've been treating teenagers with Bipolar II more often with lithium, as well as anticonvulsant drugs including Depakote, Tegretol, Trileptal, and Lamictal, and the results are promising.

The relationship between the use of selective serotonin reuptake inhibitors (SSRIs) and suicidal ideation and behaviors has received considerable attention in the media. The use of such drugs by pediatric psychiatrists/psychopharmacologists among children and teens has been of particular concern. However, there remain differences among expert psychopharmacologists and statisticians analyzing the data in the United States and England as to whether taking SSRIs in childhood or adolescence truly increases the statistical likelihood of suicidal ideas or the act of suicide. The doubt that has been cast on the subject has led pharmaceutical companies and the American Psychological Association to exhibit a warning sign in the *Physician's Desk Reference (PDR)* and the most up-to-date articles and text on the subject (i.e., "the seriously depressed child being treated with an SSRI must be monitored by parents and psychiatrists very closely while beginning SSRI treatment"). This simply means that the parents and psychiatrists must question the child directly about any feelings of self-harm or suicidal ideas. The psychiatrist must be accessible at all times, and any warning signs or symptoms on the part of the child must result in increased vigilance at the home, a change of medication, and/or possibly hospitalization.

Many scientists continue to debate the statistical meaning and correlation between increased suicidal acts and thoughts and the administration of SSRIs in children and adolescents. Experts continue to point out that many severely depressed children and adolescents, before given SSRIs, harbored suicidal thoughts, engaged in self-destructive behavior, and, at times, had made suicidal gestures.

Because of the rising rate of mental illness among young adults and college students, the National Alliance for the Mentally Ill encourages parents to start early and talk to young children about their feelings, day-to-day problems, and emotional state. Establish an open dialogue that continues into adolescence and young adulthood so the child feels comfortable sharing any personal emotions that might be symptoms of depression or hypomania. If your child has emotions or behaviors that might seem abnormal, talk to a mental health professional and seek help immediately.

AGING AND BIPOLAR II DISORDER

No one escapes the changes that come with age, and sometimes it is difficult for a physician to distinguish age-associated dementia from major depression or Bipolar II depression. Still, while major depression and bipolar disorder can coexist with dementia and Alzheimer's disease, it is atypical to diagnose Bipolar II for the first time in elderly patients. For instance, an elderly patient may have signs of depression, which can be a symptom of bipolar disorder, or it can be a sign of a yet undiagnosed chronic or terminal illness. What's more, depression can also stem from years of alcohol or substance abuse. That is why the specialist must always take a careful look at the results of the physical examination and specific laboratory tests, as well as the patient's extensive medical and family history, to see if the symptoms are caused by a medication or even age-related dementia or Alzheimer's disease. While we rarely diagnose Bipolar II disorder for the first time in those over age 65, we must look for possible medical reasons beyond the symptoms of depression or hypomania to make an accurate diagnosis.

Sometimes older patients present with symptoms of

depression when, in fact, the feelings are a reactive mood to a loss unrelated to the depression associated with Bipolar II disorder. As an example, let's look at John, a 68-year-old retired businessman who had been extremely successful in the retail industry. After his wife died of a sudden heart attack at age 64, John became sullen, withdrawn, and very forgetful. His daughter, a guidance counselor at a Long Island high school, encouraged him to have a physical examination to make sure nothing was seriously wrong. After the exam and routine laboratory blood tests, John's primary care physician told him that he probably had the very earliest signs of dementia or Alzheimer's disease. Understandably disturbed, John began to feel hopeless, ignoring his daily hygiene, eating infrequently, and sleeping most of the daytime hours. He missed appointments with former business colleagues and even failed to show up for his youngest granddaughter's birthday party. Concerned about the dramatic changes in her dad's behavior, John's daughter urged him to come see me when she suspected that his low mood, forgetfulness, and lack of interest in things around him (including his grandchildren, whom he usually loved to spend time with) might be symptoms of depression, rather than dementia.

As I evaluated John, I considered whether he might have had Bipolar II disorder in younger years, recognizing that he had been a very successful and highly productive entrepreneur before retirement, which could be suggestive of hypomania. But John said he had never felt "low" until after he sold his business and his wife of 44 years died. I then suspected that John might be suffering with mild depression, which could be reactive in nature, considering the tremendous losses he had recently experienced. Depression is common in older adults and may be the result of grief and bereavement due to the loss of a loved one, a home, a job, or income.

I prescribed a low-dose antidepressant along with talk therapy so John could start to understand his emotionally triggered low mood and, hopefully, start to make some new goals for his retirement years. When John returned to my office 6 months later for a follow-up visit, he was a different man—full of ideas, positive about life, and planning to build a retirement home in the woods in Vermont, where he had fond boyhood memories of vacationing in the summer. He stopped the antidepressant after a year and has adjusted to his new retirement and lifestyle. He continues to check in with me every 6 months to assess his mood.

Psychiatrists usually diagnose bipolar disorder in younger patients (early twenties) when they first notice the dramatic moodswings of major depression and hypomania. Still, the process of making the diagnosis in an elderly person—taking the patient and family medical history, conducting a physical examination, and collecting laboratory findings—is no different from doing the same with adults of any age, as I discussed in chapter 7.

Sometimes an elderly person exhibits signs and symptoms of Bipolar II that turn out to be the result of a medication he or she is taking for another health problem. The treatment in this instance may be to reduce the dosage or even change the medication. Elderly adults often require lower doses of medications than younger adults because of the decline in renal clearance and volume associated with aging. This means that a standard adult dose of medication may not clear the elderly person's body quickly enough, resulting in higher medication levels in the blood that could become toxic. On the other hand, the patient's symptoms could be the result of previously diagnosed Bipolar II disorder that is poorly treated or has been left untreated; or, as is often the case, the patient may have stopped the bipolar medications thinking she was well, and the depressive and hypomanic symptoms flared again. A psychiatrist must be thorough and thoughtful as he or she determines the patient's current psychiatric disturbance and then treats the problem with the most effective medication with the fewest side effects.

If I suspect that an elderly patient has Bipolar II, I use the same multiphase diagnosis/treatment process that I discussed in chapter 7, prescribing proper medication, if needed. I then refer the patient to a licensed social worker, occupational therapist, or geriatric psychologist to help him or her separate and then deal with the various environmental factors (social, economic, emotional, and medical) that usually contribute to the severity of the bipolar mood disorder in older patients.

Many elderly adults with bipolar disorder have lengthy histories of comorbid psychiatric problems such as alcoholism and drug abuse that can confound their bipolar problem at that stage in the life cycle. For instance, if Bipolar II has been misdiagnosed and/or untreated for decades, the elderly adult may have experienced a lifetime of problems such as multiple divorces, a decline in household income, no permanent residence, poor medical care, and even jail or imprisonment. To treat an elderly Bipolar II patient with all of these coexisting problems is most difficult for a psychiatrist or psychopharmacologist, and doctors usually call in a licensed social worker or psychologist for referral because these professionals are skilled in helping patients pull their lives back together.

Some of the signs and symptoms of Bipolar I or II disorder mimic age-associated dementia, including its depression, confusion, insomnia, grandiosity, or hallucinations. We see these symptoms in Alzheimer's disease, as well, and oftentimes physicians get confused while trying to make the diagnosis. However, the patient with Alzheimer's disease also has other more noticeable symptoms, including difficulty performing familiar tasks, problems with abstract thinking such as balancing a checkbook, impaired memory and forgetfulness, an inability to follow simple commands, and problems with language and communication, among others.

Often, it's a family member who must be proactive in bringing the elderly person's change in behavior to the attention of a physician. The daughter of one of my elderly Bipolar II patients was concerned when she found an "old fully cooked chicken" in her mother's kitchen cabinet and a carton of eggs stored neatly on a shelf in the warm laundry room, next to the detergent. She said that her mother had been forgetful lately and had even forgotten where she was several times while shopping, and a police officer had driven her home. As these were not new aspects of the Bipolar II disorder, I urged the woman to make an appointment for her mother to see a neurologist. Within weeks, the neurologist diagnosed the elderly woman with Alzheimer's disease, which co-occurred with her Bipolar II.

Currently, there is *no* definitive diagnostic test for dementia or Alzheimer's disease. When I suspect this in a patient, I order a complete neurological evaluation at Columbia. For an Alzheimer's patient who has coexisting major depression, dysthymia, or bipolar disorder, psychiatrists usually prescribe antidepressants or mood stabilizers, which can cause an immediate improvement in the mood. However, the antidepressant or mood stabilizer does *not* "cure" the Alzheimer's disease or the other varied symptoms, as the brain disease rapidly progresses until it takes over. True, some patients may function better temporarily on antidepressants or mood stabilizers, but the memory defect and other symptoms of dementia will still be obvious to family and friends. We often prescribe the same antipsychotics used for bipolar disorder to decrease the agitation and the insomnia associated with dementia and Alzheimer's disease.

Bipolar depression is not to be confused with late life depression that coexists with many common medical problems during that period of life, including cardiovascular disease, diabetes, and cancer, among others. Many times patients with underlying diseases such as prostate or pancreatic cancer present with depression as the only symptom. The doctor later discovers the cancer during the physical exam and blood work. Patients with chronic obstructive pulmonary disease (COPD), including emphysema and chronic bronchitis, may have depression and difficulty sleeping. That is why it is imperative to see a medical doctor immediately for a complete evaluation if you or a family member has signs and symptoms of depression. The mood change may be a red alert to a serious health problem.

For instance, 69-year-old Robert came to my office with symptoms of low mood. I ordered a physical examination and prostate-specific antigen (PSA) test, which measures the level of PSA in the blood. PSA is a biological marker or tumor marker

For Those with Bipolar II and Their Family Members

- No matter what the stage in life—childhood or adolescence, young adulthood, or elderly adult—Bipolar II has the power to destroy, or it can be restrained and methodically managed using a combination of effective and safe medications, psychotherapy, and lifestyle measures such as getting quality sleep and managing stress.
- There are specific times when patients cannot take any medication for their bipolar mood disorder, such as during pregnancy or breastfeeding, as the bipolar medications can be harmful to the baby. If you are pregnant or planning to become pregnant, it is important to work as a team with your obstetrician, mood specialist, and family members to keep your mood even during this time. You might find that psychotherapy helps to prevent exacerbations of major depression, hypomania, or mania. Talking with your mood specialist frequently, especially during times of great stress or if you are unable to sleep, might help prevent disabling moodswings.

and can help detect disease. When Robert's PSA test came in moderately elevated, I referred him to a urologist at Columbia, who later diagnosed Robert with prostate cancer. Within a week, Robert underwent surgery, which was successful in treating the cancer. When he came back to my office 2 months later, his depression had resolved.

- If your child has been diagnosed with ADHD, talk to your pediatrician about the possibility of Bipolar II disorder if you have a family history of mood disorders. Getting an accurate diagnosis and the right treatment for a child or adolescent with Bipolar II disorder is necessary to ensure good quality of life. If the medications are not helping your child's moodswings, talk to a pediatric psychopharmacologist for a more thorough evaluation and proper treatment.
- If you are over 65 and have been diagnosed with a mood disorder, check with your internist or geriatric specialist to see if it's being treated effectively. Some medications work differently in older adults. You may need a change in dosage or in medication to feel your best.
- Though it is an increasingly common mood disorder, with proper education, Bipolar II disorder can be highly recognized, quickly diagnosed, easily discussed, and managed in such a way that the patient and his or her family can have a most successful life.

CHAPTER 10

STAY-WELL STRATEGIES

If you have Bipolar II, you must be your own mental health guardian. This means making informed decisions regarding early recognition of warning signs of an impending episode and also being compliant with regular doctor's visits to monitor your mood and medications.

While treating Bipolar II disorder is critical, especially in the early stages when treatment is most effective, there is a compelling case supported by a host of scientific data that the *prevention of further episodes* altogether should be the utmost goal. Having diagnosed and treated bipolar patients for decades, in this last chapter, I will give you some simple but effective "stay-well" strategies that can help you become more aware of this illness and protect yourself and your loved ones from the devastation of major depression or out-of-control hypomania or mania.

STRATEGY #1: MONITOR YOUR MOOD

Your doctor will not know how you are feeling if you do not monitor your mood. I cannot tell you how many patients call my office only when their family members insist that they are out of control, with their mood having escalated to a state of hypomanic elation or severe depression. At this point, the patient and his or her family members are desperate for help. Why patients wait until the last moment to seek treatment, when it's much more difficult to manage the out-of-control mood, continues to challenge and frustrate me. However, I've observed that most patients with Bipolar II resist treatment for fear of dampening the exuberant energy and creativity. After all, most of my patients and their families usually know how Bipolar II disorder manifests itself in mood and behavior and are aware that early treatment usually stops impending serious episodes.

I believe that it is important for anyone questioning their psychological well-being to rate their moods and behavior from time to time. For that reason, I developed the following Self-Rating Mood Scale for my own patients to use. After charting their moods for several weeks, many patients have called my office to get treatment when they noticed their daily mood leaning toward depression or hypomania. By using this chart each day over a period of a few weeks, you can become more aware of how your moodswings feel as they approach—both the descents into depression and the ascents into hypomania. You may want to copy pages 234 and 235 and post them where you can see them as a constant reminder to check your mood daily. Review the scale every day for 1 week before breakfast because, as I discussed on pages 96 and 97, Bipolar II patients usually have the greatest peak of their diurnal depression in the morning hours. Place a mark in the chart where you feel your mood most closely correlates with the definitions given on the chart. At the end of the week, observe the patterns of your moods from Monday to Sunday, as well as any dramatic changes. (Note that both delusional psychotic depression and manic psychosis are medical emergencies and require immediate help.)

Dr. Fieve's Self-Rating Mood Scale

	M	T	W	TH	F	SAT	SUN
+4							
+3							
+2							
+1							
0							
-1							
-2							
-3							
-4							

-4   (Delusional Psychotic Depression) You have delusions and hallucinations in addition to the symptoms of major depression. You are experiencing total withdrawal or extreme agitation. (This is a medical emergency.)

-3   (Major Depression) You have a depressed mood with loss of interest or pleasure in ordinary activities. You have loss of energy, disturbed patterns of eating and sleeping, and feelings of hopelessness. You have difficulty concentrating or making decisions and no interest in sex. You may have suicidal feelings.

-2 (Dysthymic) You are mildly depressed with low self-confidence, low energy, and loss of interest and pleasure in activities you normally enjoy. Your daily mood is pessimistic. (If the low mood persists most days for 2 years, see your doctor or mental health professional for an evaluation. There are medications that can safely and quickly treat dysthymia.)

-1 (Hypothymic) You are reasonably well adjusted and function adequately, but are low-key and slightly withdrawn. You may be a follower rather than a leader. You smile infrequently, work efficiently, and are conscientious. You often have obsessive-compulsive or perfectionist personality traits.

---

0 (Normal) You have no symptoms of depression or hypomanic elation. You function well in social, professional, and interpersonal areas. You have appropriate reactions to daily disappointments and successes.

+1 (Hyperthymic) You are highly energetic, motivated, and productive and extremely successful. You are sociable but sometimes irritable. You are often a leader in all walks of life and usually well liked. You may need only 5 to 6 hours of sleep a night and do not seek therapy.

+2 (Hypomanic) Your predominant mood is highly energetic, expansive, and elevated. You are full of innovative ideas and projects. You often get angry when crossed, and at times you are irritating to others. You have a strong sex drive and compulsively spend money, travel, and talk. You require only 3 to 5 hours of sleep and often make poor judgments and engage in risky behaviors that may lead to legal consequences. Hypomania may be highly beneficial, as in you may exhibit Bipolar IIB, or it can be detrimental.

+3 (Manic) You are highly elated and overactive, and you cannot stop talking. You need little or even no sleep and are highly distractible, irritable, and angry. You have racing thoughts and rage attacks when crossed. You exhibit paranoid ideas, extremely poor judgment, and depressive features and may require hospitalization.

+4 (Manic Psychosis) You are incoherent, belligerent, and out of control. You may be violent or paranoid with psychotic delusions and hallucinations. You exhibit risk-taking behaviors with painful consequences. Depressive features may be present. (This is a medical emergency. Hospitalization is essential.)

STRATEGY #2: SEEK PSYCHOTHERAPY

The role of psychotherapy in mood disorders is to help a person develop appropriate and workable coping strategies to deal with everyday stressors and to increase medication compliance. I was trained initially as a psychoanalyst at Columbia and later as a researcher who evaluates whether a specific treatment works. From my years of experience working with Bipolar II patients, I believe that psychotherapy is meaningful for some patients in whom depression is first relieved by antidepressants. For example, psychotherapy has been proven useful with dysthymia, alone or with antidepressant treatment. Subsequent adjunctive psychotherapy may aid the patient taking an antidepressant to socially readjust to problems of living.

Because Bipolar II disorder is a lifelong disease with a risk of recurrent episodes, it is important to assess the psychosocial factors that might help patients improve functioning and compliance in keeping their doctors' appointments where blood levels of lithium and anticonvulsive medications will be monitored. Of the patients who come to my consulting practice, about 80 percent have already been treated with various types of psychiatric medications by anywhere from 1 to 10 previous private or clinical psychiatrists or general practitioners. Many have had long courses of psychotherapy from which they report little to no benefit as their moodswings have continued unabated. Some findings indicate that the average length of compliance with mood stabilizers after bipolar patients are treated for the first time is only 2 months.[1] After this period of time, many Bipolar II patients feel well and think they are "cured," so they abruptly discontinue the medication. They may live quite normally for a short or longer (weeks to months) period of time— until the illness flares again. Psychological intervention can provide patients with methods that will increase their awareness of Bipolar II triggers and early warning signs. They can then call their doctors, who should immediately intervene with appropriate mood-stabilizing medications, thus minimizing the risk of full relapse. In most cases, it is important that the psychotherapist performing these services is trained in the area of Bipolar II disorders and works closely with the psychiatrist. The psychotherapist in my New York office is trained in basic psychopharmacologic treatment.

Some psychotherapy options for treating Bipolar II are described in the following sections.

Individual Counseling

This is a one-on-one session with a professional therapist (either a doctor with a PhD or DSci, a clinical social worker, a nurse practitioner, or a physician's assistant) with experience in bipolar disorders in which individual problem areas are addressed. The session may include specific help with acceptance of the diagnosis, education about bipolar disorder, ways to identify the warning signs of an episode, and intervention strategies to manage Bipolar II triggers so you may be able to avoid a major episode.

Because life's stressors can exacerbate a depressive or hypomanic mood episode, one-to-one sessions can help the resistant patient with bipolar disorder to identify stressors, as well as increase coping skills and overall resilience. As discussed earlier in chapter 4, adequate sleep is especially important in Bipolar II disorder since poor sleep may precipitate a depressive or hypomanic episode. Working with a therapist, patients can learn to identify stumbling blocks to sleep and develop healthy patterns of activity and social involvement, thereby influencing their overall quality of life. The adjunctive therapeutic sessions focus on compliance with regular office appointments, taking prescribed doses of medications, and obtaining blood medication levels, when needed.

Family Counseling

As illustrated with the myriad stories throughout this book, bipolar disorder extends beyond the patient and can affect the entire family. Family members often have to cope with the patient's wide and often unexpected moodswings, wild spending sprees or impulsivity during the hypomania, or extreme irritability, haughtiness, and depression. While family members may have the best of intentions, without professional guidance, they sometimes inadvertently make things worse.

Families are frequently involved in outpatient therapy as they become educated about the various symptoms of Bipolar II disorder and work with the therapist and patient to learn how to recognize early warning signs of an impending episode. Recent findings suggest that these sessions may be valuable treatment components, adding significant benefit to medication compliance and lifestyle and sleep management.

Family meetings are also beneficial for helping everyone deal with the stress of an emotional illness and allowing the patient and family members to openly discuss grievances without placing blame.

Group Counseling

I sometimes find that there is no one who can better understand Bipolar II disorder than another person with the same illness. Group sessions allow for the sharing of feelings and the development of effective coping strategies. Karin, a 40-year-old woman with Bipolar II, found tremendous support in group counseling. "I feel emotionally stronger now," she said. "My group sessions meet every Wednesday night and give me the opportunity to share my problems and successes with others. Somehow, the anger and resentment I had about this disorder is alleviated when I hear how successful others who participate in group therapy are in managing their medications and their lives."

The give-and-take at group sessions is often the most productive way to change how you think about your illness and improve your ability to cope with life's challenges and difficulties.

Therapy for Emotional and/or Behavioral Issues

For the treatment of the emotional and behavioral concerns that arise with Bipolar II disorder, Cognitive Behavioral Therapy, Dialectic Behavioral Therapy, Interpersonal Psychotherapy, and Social Rhythm Therapy are widely used interventions. These therapies focus on helping the patient identify early warning signs, interrupt unrealistic thought patterns and perceptions, and change potentially destructive behaviors.

Through my experience working with patients, I have seen that people with Bipolar II disorder tend to have similar problems, even though the structures of families are different and individual manifestations of depression or hypomania vary. For example, I have patients with Bipolar II who have severe episodes of depression that can make them despondent if they are unmedicated. I have other patients who experience milder depressions, more like dysthymia, who continue to function in their daily living activities but at a slower pace, preferring to ride out the mild depression with no medications at all.

Many people with bipolar disorder feel frustrated at having to depend on medications to control their moods. These medications can affect sleep, appetite, body weight, and sexual performance. One patient told me that he was going to seek a divorce because of sexual problems resulting from his medication. "I feel useless," he said. "I cannot function the way a normal man should, and I have no way of solving it." (After he told me about this problem, I prescribed Viagra [sildenafil citrate], a safe medication that restored his erectile function, and his marital relationship with his wife is now back to normal.)

Fear becomes a great issue with bipolar disorder as people question what might happen in the future. Patients often ask me, "Will my Bipolar II disorder worsen as I get older?" or "Will I be forced to quit my job?" or "What if the medications stop working to control my symptoms?"

I realize that it is not pleasurable to live with any chronic illness—physical or mental. At their most frustrated moments, some of my patients have said that a "life with Bipolar II disorder is like no life at all." Untreated, the Bipolar II patients' problems and fears are real and are often devastating to their outlook on life and daily living. That's why talk therapy to deal with the emotional and behavioral issues becomes crucial for most patients.

Cognitive Behavioral Therapy. The tendency with Bipolar II disorder is to see yourself, the world around you, and the future in a negative way, such that it often leads to depression. Cognitive Behavioral Therapy (CBT) is a short-term, goal-oriented intervention that focuses on how the patient's negative misperceptions and views about himself, the world around him, and the future precede and influence behavior and trigger anxiety and depression.

With CBT, the therapist works with you to isolate ways in which you might misperceive information and then uses various techniques to help you change these dysfunctional thoughts and subsequent behavior. Some studies indicate that longer-term CBT may significantly improve the outcome of those with Bipolar II disorder, particularly if they are also compliant with medication, thereby reducing the severity and/or number of episodes. I prescribe CBT during my initial consultation with patients for 12 to 16 successive weekly sessions, at which time and periodically, the therapist and I meet to re-evaluate the overall progress and treatment process.

Dialectic Behavioral Therapy. With Dialectic Behavioral Therapy (DBT), patients learn to examine and validate their current emotions and behaviors, especially those that have a negative impact on their lives. The therapist then helps the patient learn problem-solving skills to help him or her deal with life's problems both personally and socially. While DBT was originally designed for those with borderline personality disorder, it has been my experience that some patients with Bipolar II disorder who undergo DBT with medications have fewer suicide attempts and less hospitalization.

Interpersonal Psychotherapy. This three-part, time-limited therapy is specifically designed to help patients alleviate mild depression. During the first one to three sessions, the psychotherapist takes a psychiatric history and an interpersonal inventory that focuses on the patient's psychosocial problems. The middle phase of Interpersonal Psychotherapy focuses on the problems of the present (rather than the past) through a series of strategies designed to help the patient cope with grief, interpersonal conflicts, role transitions, and inadequate social skills. During the final phase, the therapist helps the patient learn to recognize and cope with symptoms of depression that might appear in the future.

Various studies have shown that Interpersonal Psychotherapy is an effective therapy for some forms of mild depression (dysthymia) even without drugs. This is important because there are many instances in which depressed patients cannot take a drug. Some people are simply not responsive to drugs, and others experience side effects that range from uncomfortable to extremely serious. Others can have medical problems that make taking an antidepressant or mood-stabilizing drug problematic or even toxic (for instance, in pregnancy). Others simply do not want to take them. The best results, however, especially during the mild phase of a Bipolar II depression, usually come from the combination of Cognitive Behavioral Therapy or Interpersonal Psychotherapy with an antidepressant medication.

Interpersonal and Social Rhythm Therapy. This one-on-one therapy combines Interpersonal Psychotherapy with behavioral techniques to help patients learn how to diminish interpersonal problems, stay compliant to their medication regimen, and regularize their lifestyle habits, such as getting plenty of sleep, learning to cope with chronic stress, and avoiding excess alcohol.

It is thought that a disruption in social rhythms, which are life events that can be either positive or negative, might disturb the body's circadian rhythms and the sleep-wake cycle. Because individuals with Bipolar II disorder have a genetic vulnerability to alterations in circadian rhythm and sleep-wake cycle abnormalities that may contribute to symptoms of the illness (see pages 93 to 95), Interpersonal and Social Rhythm Therapy is often beneficial. In research findings, Ellen Frank, PhD, director of the depression and manic depression prevention program at Western Psychiatric Institute and Clinic, and colleagues at the University of Pittsburgh School of Medicine concluded that this type of therapy may play a key role in improving overall function and long-term remission in those with bipolar disorder.

STRATEGY #3: STRENGTHEN YOUR SUPPORT NETWORK

While you cannot control your diagnosis of Bipolar II disorder, there are some things you can control. You can seek or create a positive support system for yourself. Whether your social network stems from your spouse, family members, close friends, co-workers, religious organizations, or community groups, support is available.

While not everyone in your support network can be there for you all the time, it's important to consider the different types of support that are most helpful for someone with a chronic illness, including:

- **Emotional support.** Someone you trust with your most intimate thoughts, including hopes and fears. This could be your spouse, a close friend, or a health care worker.
- **Social support.** Someone you enjoy being with to share life experiences. This might be a family member, colleague, close friend, or neighbor with common interests.

- **Informational support.** Someone you can ask for advice on major decisions. Many people in professional life look at these individuals as mentors. This could be your doctor, attorney, counselor, or religious leader.
- **Practical support.** Someone who will help you out in a pinch. Sometimes, neighbors or co-workers are in this category.

Social Support Helps You Feel Accepted

If you've ever had a severe episode, you know how important it is to have trusted family members and friends to lean on. Ongoing encouragement and support are also needed after a person starts treatment. There are findings showing that the availability of social support systems increases the chances of employment in patients with bipolar disorder compared with those patients without tangible support.[2]

Social Support Helps You to Be Resilient

Research on stress-resistant personality traits has identified keys to staying healthy, including the following:

- Involvement in work or other tasks that have great meaning
- The ability to relate well to others
- The ability to interact in a strong social network[3]

Personality resilience or hardiness is a pattern of attitudes and actions that helps in changing life's stressors from possible disasters into growth opportunities. In a recent article published in *American Psychologist,* study author Salvatore R. Maddi, PhD, professor of psychology at the University of California, Irvine, and founder of the Hardiness Institute, describes hardy attitudes as having the motivation to face stressors accurately (rather than to deny or catastrophize them). Dr. Maddi contends that this courage and motivation lead to coping by problem solving rather than avoiding and/or interacting with others, by giving and getting assistance and encouragement rather than by striking out at others.[4]

Social Support Keeps You Accountable

Social support helps those with Bipolar II keep their doctors' appointments, avoid self-medicating with alcohol or drugs, and control their lifestyle habits to avoid an episode. Led by David Miklowitz, PhD, researchers at the University of Colorado at Boulder concluded in a yearlong study that patients who received medication and an experimental family-focused treatment program had fewer episodes of Bipolar II disorder as well as longer delays before relapses than those who received medication alone and standard community treatment.[5] In my practice, I have found that social support helps the patient accept warning signs of an impending episode instead of ignoring them. For example, your spouse may comment that you have not been getting enough sleep, and perhaps you should call your doctor. Because you know that loss of sleep might precede a hypomanic or depressive episode, this supportive "nudge" can alert you and cause you to seek early intervention with a doctor's visit and proper medications. Because of a supportive family member being aware of your lifestyle habits, you may modulate your moods and medication before having a relapse. By avoiding relapse, you can stay positive, improve your family relationships, and be a productive person at home and in the workplace.

Support Groups Offer Encouragement

Support groups such as those sponsored by the National Depressive and Manic Depressive Association (NDMDA), the National Alliance for the Mentally Ill (NAMI), the Foundation for Mood Disorders (FMD), and the National Mental Health

Association (NMHA) are geared toward meeting the unique needs of those with Bipolar II disorder. Although support groups are not psychotherapy groups amd instead are often educational, they do provide patients and families with a safe and accepting environment to vent their frustrations, share their personal stories, and receive comfort and encouragement from one another. In many such groups, the latest medications are discussed and coping suggestions are shared amongst members. Assurance is given that someone else knows what you are going through as people share their struggles in living with Bipolar II disorder. After joining a support group, you may realize that the best experts on bipolar disorder are those men and women who live with it daily, although it still remains critically important to talk with your doctor before trying any treatment suggested by other patients in the group.

Families and friends can also benefit from support groups offered by these organizations. Talk to your doctor or check with your local mental health association for more information.

If you have no time to attend a support group, you can find support in the privacy of your own home or office via the Internet. You can "chat" on message boards or exchange e-mail with those in different states or even foreign countries who may have gone through the same problems that you are experiencing.

The pressures of living with a chronic emotional illness can be overwhelming, but it does not have to be this way, if you seek support from others. Ask your doctor to recommend professional help and resources, including professional counselors, psychologists, and support groups with other patients who have Bipolar II disorder. Send away for government pamphlets and brochures using the addresses in the back of this book, or go online and find a support group on the Internet.

Support from others can help you realize that you are *not* alone in dealing with Bipolar II disorder. This support can give you new confidence as you learn to manage the illness and handle the daily challenges in a reasonable manner.

STRATEGY #4: RESOLVE SLEEP PROBLEMS

I discussed sleep and its relationship to bipolar disorder in chapter 4. Still, I want to reiterate the importance of getting restful sleep to avoid serious episodes of depression or hypomania. Comprehensive studies point to sleep habits as possible indicators of whether a Bipolar II patient is likely to relapse or remain in remission. Staying on a regular sleep schedule may help prevent rapid cycling in patients with hypomania, while perturbations in circadian rhythms may be early markers of impending relapse.[6] In my own practice, I have documented sleep problems in many of my Bipolar II patients even between acute episodes of depression or hypomania.

Evaluate your sleep hygiene to make sure your body is totally prepared for rest. It's difficult to sleep when you have lights on, the television blaring, and your laptop computer on the nightstand. Some simple suggestions that might help you rest include eliminating caffeine from your diet, exercising regularly during the morning or afternoon hours but not near bedtime, and eating your last meal at least 3 hours before you get in bed. Sometimes a snack that is high in carbohydrates such as cereal and milk or a bagel helps to induce sleep because it boosts the levels of serotonin (see page 101), the chemical messenger in the brain that regulates mood, appetite, and sleep. Make sure your bedroom is quiet and dark. Consider using earplugs, which you can purchase at any supermarket or drugstore, and install black-out shades, found at any home fix-it store, to keep outside lights from disrupting your sleep. Some individuals who are sensitive to sound find that "white noise" machines help lull them to sleep. These are available online and at most department stores.

Talk to your doctor if you have difficulty falling asleep or maintaining sleep. There are new nonaddictive medications available that can help resolve sleep problems. Also, Cognitive Behavioral Therapy has been shown in recent clinical trials to be a helpful adjunct treatment for patients with Bipolar II who have impaired sleep efficiency, or anxiety and fears about poor sleep.[7]

STRATEGY #5: FIND MEDICATIONS THAT WORK

I see many patients with Bipolar II who have a lifetime history of going on and off medications. Or they think they can "hang in there" a few more days until the depression or hypomania passes. Most of the time, these patients will take medication for about 2 months and then feel much better with their newly controlled moods. Thinking they are now "well," they stop taking the medications. Then in a few weeks to months, they invariably call my office asking to see me again to refill the old prescription.

To avoid swinging too high or falling too low with Bipolar II disorder, it is important to find the most effective medication that works for you, in the dosages that work best for you. You must take the medication as prescribed, especially when you feel "well," for prevention of future episodes.

Bipolar II disorder does not go away. But you can take precautionary measures to keep it from totally disrupting your life should it reappear. Staying on medication will help prevent unexpected moodswings, so that you can remain productive and active. If you feel that your medication is not working or is accompanied by too many side effects, call and see your doctor immediately to resolve the problem. With all of the new medications continually being discovered to treat Bipolar II disorder, your doctor or psychiatrist can help you find the right drug in the right dosage that will help you achieve that perfect mood balance.

STRATEGY #6: CHECK YOUR ATTITUDE

No matter what your diagnosis, perhaps the most important factor in gaining control over your bipolar disorder is realizing that the illness is not your fault. Nothing you did—or did not do—caused the bipolar disorder. I make it clear to all of my patients that if they stay on their medications and keep their doctor's visits, whereby their moods, behaviors, and blood medication levels (if indicated) are monitored, they will most likely see excellent results. Having a positive attitude alone may make the difference between being able to get up and go to work each day or staying home alone and living an isolated life void of social support and activity.

When my patients have difficulty accepting their illness, I urge them to consider how someone with a resilient personality would handle the situation. We know that resilient people have fewer and less severe illnesses and cope better than those who are not as resilient. How can you make yourself more resilient? You might:

- Maintain a sense of control. This means an ability to face future situations with determination rather than helplessness.
- Be a survivor. When problems happen, find ways to take action and prepare to endure them and see them through.
- Stay involved in life. Don't allow yourself to become withdrawn and pull away from family and close friends.
- Make a commitment to stick with healthy habits. While a healthful diet and regular exercise cannot "cure" bipolar disorder, positive lifestyle habits are important for staying healthy and avoiding other ailments.
- Keep your activity at the highest level within your personal limits. It is important to get involved in a local church or religious organization. Volunteer to serve on neighborhood committees. Be a mentor or tutor in your neighborhood school.
- Be determined. Do not let your bipolar disorder stop your personal and career goals.
- Look for areas of growth and opportunity. Though you may still have some moodswings, there is a world of opportunity for you to use your talents and energy.

For Those with Bipolar II and Their Family Members

- Monitor your mood each day using the chart on pages 234 and 235. If you notice your mood swinging higher or lower than normal for at least 3 or 4 days up to 2 weeks, call your doctor for treatment and/or psychotherapy. Family members should also stay aware of the person's mood swings and alert the patient or the doctor if there is a dramatic or consistent change in mood.

- Stay actively involved in your job, religious and community organizations, and recreational activities. I find that too many patients are hesitant to become involved in outside organizations or activities because of the stigma of having a mood disorder. But social support can help you feel accepted and even improve your sense of self-worth.

- Quality sleep is vital in keeping moods balanced. If you have difficulty falling asleep or maintaining sleep, try to make changes in your nighttime routine. You can try earplugs, a sleep mask, black-out shades, and even white noise to help decrease the outside stimulation that may be keeping you revved up. Talk to your doctor about your sleep difficulties if they continue to be a problem.

- Psychotherapy can help you to develop appropriate and workable coping strategies to handle daily stress. I believe that family therapy is best, especially with a newly diagnosed patient or a patient who is not compliant to taking the necessary medication.

- Belief is crucial in overcoming the obstacles Bipolar II disorder can throw in your path. Most of my patients who were once totally crippled by depressive symptoms return to exciting careers and active social lives when they finally accept the chronic illness and become committed to taking daily medications (if needed) to prevent further episodes.

ACKNOWLEDGMENTS

The task of increasing public awareness and improving the diagnosis and treatment of Bipolar II disorder with its intriguing hypomania and major depression is truly a team effort. Without the ongoing support of my family, friends, colleagues, patients, and other professionals, this book would not have been possible.

First, there would be *no book* without my collaborator, Debra Fulghum Bruce, PhD, whose writing ability and understanding of Bipolar II and related disorders made the completion of this comprehensive book possible. When a new idea struck me, I immediately reached Deb on the phone to share my thoughts with her. For her energy, enthusiasm, and willingness to work with me, I am most grateful. I especially thank her for being a true professional. Whatever challenges we faced, she remained calm, focused, and flexible.

I also want to thank John Berg, a doctoral student in psychology at Emory University in Atlanta, Georgia, and Britt Berg, MS, clinical research coordinator at Emory University Medical School, working under Debra Bruce, for their hours of journal research that helped to substantiate this project.

I express heartfelt thanks to my personal assistant, Karon Gilbey. Karon's untiring support in communications, computer proficiency, administrative skills, and Bipolar II research allowed me to focus on creating the book.

I am also indebted to Monica Gilbert for her administrative leadership and her extraordinary office and computer skills employed at my New York City private practice while I dedicated many nights and weekends to research and writing.

To Margarite Howe, my writer assistant for my first book, *Moodswing*, I cannot thank her enough for the contributions she made in the early stages of writing *Bipolar II*.

I am indebted to Vanessa Fieve Willett, managing director of Fieve Clinical Services, whose drug trials over the past 6 years helped produce several groundbreaking bipolar and depressive medications recently released, i.e. Lamictal, and to Lara Fieve Portela, principal research coordinator at Fieve Clinical Services, for her careful evaluation of data in clinical trials following her years of extensive training at Pfizer and for her humanitarian approach as managing director of my private practice.

To my agent, Beth Vesel, who proposed the idea of writing *Bipolar II* as a sequel to my first book, *Moodswing*.

To my Rodale editors—Stephanie Tade, Jennifer Kushnier, Andrea Au Levitt, Mariska van Aalst and Zachary Greenwald—I am most grateful for their professional skills in editing this book.

APPENDIX:
RESOURCES

GENERAL RESOURCE LIST

Following is a list of organizations that can provide additional information about and/or assistance for bipolar disorder and other psychiatric health topics.

American Psychiatric Association (APA)
1000 Wilson Boulevard, Suite 1825
Arlington, VA 22209-3901
Phone: 703-907-7300
www.psych.org

American Psychological Association
750 1st Street, NE
Washington, DC 20002-4242
Phone: 202-336-5510
Toll-free: 800-374-2721
www.apa.org

Center for Mental Health Services
Substance Abuse and Mental Health Services Administration
Room 12-105, Parklawn Building
Rockville, MD 20857
Phone: 301-443-8956
Fax: 301-443-9050
www.samhsa.gov

Child and Adolescent Bipolar Foundation
1187 Wilmette Avenue
PMB 331
Wilmette, IL 60091
Phone: 847-256-8525
Fax: 847-920-9498
www.bpkids.org

Depression and Bipolar Support Alliance (DBSA)
730 North Franklin Street, Suite 501
Chicago, IL 60610-7224
Phone: 312-642-0049
Fax: 312-642-7243
www.DBSAlliance.org

Depression and Related Affective Disorders Association (DRADA)
2330 West Joppa Road, Suite 100
Lutherville, MD 21093
Phone: 410-583-2919
E-mail: drada@jhmi.edu
www.drada.org

Foundation for Mood Disorders
952 Fifth Avenue, Suite 6A
New York, NY 10021
Phone: 212-772-3400
Fax: 212-288-0809

National Alliance for Research on Schizophrenia and Depression (NARSAD)
60 Cutter Mill Road, Suite 404
Great Neck, NY 11021
Phone: 516-829-0091
Toll-free: 800-829-8289
E-mail: info@narsad.org
www.narsad.org

National Institute of Mental Health
6001 Executive Boulevard, Room 8184, MSC 9663
Bethesda, MD 20892-9663
Phone: 301-443-4513
Fax: 301-443-4279
Toll-free: 866-615-NIMH (6464)
TTY: 301-443-8431
E-mail: nimhinfo@nih.gov
www.nimh.nih.gov

CLINICAL TRIALS

Below is a list of Web sites where you can find out about clinical trials (both listings and information).

www.clinicaltrials.com

www.clinicaltrialssearch.org

www.fieve.com

www.fieveclinical.com

RELATED WEB SITES

General Mental Wellness

American Academy of Addiction Psychiatry
www.aaap.org

The American College of Psychiatrists
www.acpsych.org

American Foundation for Suicide Prevention
www.afsp.org

American Medical Association
www.ama-assn.org

American Psychoanalytic Association
www.apsa.org

Anxiety Disorders Association of America (ADAA)
www.adaa.org

Center for Mental Health Services
www.mentalhealth.org

The Cross Cultural Health Care Program
www.xculture.org

Healthfinder
www.healthfinder.gov

Healthfinder Español
www.healthfinder.gov/espanol/

**Madison Institute of Medicine
(information on lithium, bipolar
disorders treatment, and
obsessive compulsive disorders)**
www.miminc.org

Mental Health Liaison Group
www.mhlg.org

Misunderstood Minds
www.pbs.org/wgbh/misunderstood
minds/index.html

**Mood and Anxiety Disorders Program
(National Institute of Mental
Health)**
http://intramural.nimh.nih.gov/mood

National Alliance for the Mentally Ill
www.nami.org

**National Association of Psychiatric
Health Systems**
www.naphs.org

National Institutes of Health
www.nih.gov

National Library of Medicine
www.nlm.nih.gov

National Mental Health Association
www.nmha.org

National Suicide Prevention Lifeline
www.suicidepreventionlifeline.org

Obsessive Compulsive Foundation
www.ocfoundation.org

**Tools for Coping with a Variety of
Life's Stressors**
www.coping.org

Children and Mental Health

About Our Kids
www.aboutourkids.org

American Academy of Pediatrics
www.aap.org

Attention Deficit Disorder Resources
www.addresources.org

**Caring for Every Child's Mental Health
Campaign**
www.mentalhealth.org/child

**Center for Treatment Research on
Adolescent Drug Abuse**
www.med.miami.edu/ctrada

The Child Advocate
www.childadvocate.net

**Child and Adolescent Bipolar
Foundation**
www.cabf.org

**Children and Adults with Attention
Deficit Disorder**
www.chadd.org

The Children's Health Council
www.chconline.org

Connect for Kids
www.connectforkids.org

Families for Depression Awareness
www.familyaware.org/

**Federation of Families for Children's
Mental Health**
www.ffcmh.org

**International Association for Child
and Adolescent Psychiatry and
Allied Professions**
www.iacapap.org

ParentsMedGuide
www.parentsmedguide.org/

**SOS High School Suicide Prevention
Program**
www.mentalhealthscreening.org/sos_
highschool

**Teen Adolescent Mental Health and
Suicide Screening Initiative**
www.teenscreen.org

ENDNOTES

Preface

[1] Ronald R. Fieve, MD. *Moodswing: Dr. Fieve on Depression*, William Morrow, 1975, 2nd Edition, Bantam Dell, 1997.

Chapter 1

[1] Frederick Goodwin, MD & Kay Redfield Jamison, *Manic-Depressive Illness*, Oxford University Press, 1991.

[2] MM Weissman, RC Bland, and GJ Canino, (1996) "Cross-Depression and Bipolar Disorder," *JAMA* (4), 293–99.

[3] B Müller-Oerlinghausen, et al., (2002). "Bipolar Disorder," *Lancet* 359(9302): 241–47.

[4] AK Das, M Olfson, MJ Gameroff, et al., "Screening for Bipolar Disorder in a Primary Care Practice," *JAMA*, 2005 Feb 23; 293(8): 956–63.

[5] SW Woods, "The Economic Burden of Bipolar Disease," *J Clin Psychiatry* 2000; 61 Supp 13:38.

[6] "Living with Bipolar Disorder: How Far Have We Really Come?" National Depressive and Manic-Depressive Association. 2002.

[7] Goodwin, F.K., Fireman, B., Simon, G.E., Hunkeler, E.M.,Lee, J., Dennis R. Suicide risk in bipolar disorder during treatment with lithium and divalproex. *JAMA*. 2003; 290(11): 1467–1473.

Chapter 2

[1] W Weiten, *Psychology: Themes and Variations*. 6th ed. (Belmont, CA: Thomson and Wadsworth, 2004).

[2] Ibid.

[3] I Shiah and L Yatham, "Serotonin in Mania and in the Mechanism of Action of Mood Stabilizers: A Review of Clinical Studies," Bipolar Disorders 2(2), June 2000: 77–92. Blackwell Publishing, United Kingdom

[4] N Brunello, P Blier, L Judd, et al., "Noradrenaline in Mood and Anxiety Disorders:

Basic and Clinical Studies," International Clinical Psychopharmacology, 18(4) July 2003, 191–202. Lippincott Williams and Wilkins, US.

5 D Dunner, "Clinical Consequences of Under-Recognized Bipolar Spectrum Disorder," *Bipolar Disorders*, 2003; 5:456–63.

6 DL Dunner, V Patrick, RR Fieve, "Rapid Cycling Manic Depressive Patients," *Compr Psychiatry*, 1977 November–December; 18(6):561–66.

7 American Psychiatric Association, *Diagnostic and Statistical Manual of Mental Disorders*, 4th ed. (Washington, DC: American Psychiatric Association, 1994), pp 332.

8 *DSM-IV*, pp. 338.

9 RC Kessler, WT Chiu, O Demler, EE Walters, "Prevalence, Severity, and Comorbidity of Twelve-Month *DSM-IV* Disorders in the National Comorbidity Survey Replication (NCS-R)," *Archives of General Psychiatry*, 2005 June; 62(6):617–27.

10 DA Regier, WE Narrow, DS Rae, et al., "The De Facto Mental and Addictive Disorders Service System. Epidemiologic Catchment Area Prospective 1-Year Prevalence Rates of Disorders and Services," Archives of General Psychiatry 1993; 50(2): 85–94.

11 *DSM-IV*. page 349.

12 CJL Murray, AD Lopez, eds. *The Global Burden of Disease and Injury Series, Volume 1: A Comprehensive Assessment of Mortality and Disability from Diseases, Injuries, and Risk Factors in 1990 and Projected to 2020* (Cambridge, MA: Published by the Harvard School of Public Health on behalf of the World Health Organization and the World Bank, Harvard University Press, 1996).

13 RC Kessler, WT Chiu, O Demler, EE Walters, "Prevalence, Severity, and Cormorbidity of Twelve-Month *DSM-IV* Disorders in the National Comorbidity Survey Replication (NCS-R)," *Archives of General Psychiatry*, 2005 June; 62(6):617–27.

14 *DSM-IV*, pp. 327.

15 H Madhukar, MD Trivedi, "The Link between Depression and Physical Symptoms," *Prim Care Companion J Clin Psychiatry*, 2004; 6(suppl 1): 12–16.

16 DSM-IV, pp. 362.

17 LM Arnold, "Gender Differences in Bipolar Disorder," *Psychiatr Clin North Am*, 2003 September; 26(3):595–620.

Chapter 3

1 SG Simpson, SE Folstein, DA Meyers, et al., "Bipolar II: The Most Common Bipolar Phenotype?" *Am J Psychiatry*, 1993 June; 150(6): 901–3.

2 KD Chang, H Steiner, and TA Ketter, "Psychiatric Phenomenology of Child and Adolescent Bipolar Offspring," *J Am Acad Child Adolesc Psychiatry*, 2000 April; 39(4): 453–60.

3 KD Chang, C Blasey, TA Ketter, and H Steiner, "Family Environment of Children and Adolescents with Bipolar Parents," *Bipolar Disord*, 2001; 2:68–72.

4 "Judge Not..." Psychology Today July–August 1997. http://cms.psychologytoday.com/articles/pto-19970701-000027.html.

5 S Wachtler, *After the Madness: A Judge's Own Prison Memoir*. (New York: Random House, 1997).

6 JE Call, "A Prominent Judge Goes to Prison." Legal Studies Forum Volume 25,

Nos 3 & 4 (2001). Tarlton Law Library. The University of Texas at Austin. http://tarlton.law.utexas.edu/lpop/etext/lsf/call25.htm#10.

[7] F Stallone, DL Dunner, J Ahearn, and RR Fieve, "Statistical Predictions of Suicide in Depressives," *Compr Psychiatry*, 1980 September–October; 21(5): 381–87.

[8] KD Chang, H Steiner, and TA Ketter, "Psychiatric Phenomenology of Child and Adolescent Bipolar Offspring," *J Am Acad Child Adolesc Psychiatry*, 2000 April; 39(4): 453–60.

[9] JM Allen, RW Lam, RA Remick, and AD Sadovnick, "Depressive Symptoms and Family History in Seasonal and Nonseasonal Mood Disorders," *Am J Psychiatry*, 1993; 150:443–48.

[10] G Perugi, HS Akiskal, "The Soft Bipolar Spectrum Redefined: Focus on the Cyclothymic, Anxious-Sensitive, Impulse-Dyscontrol, and Binge-Eating Connection in Bipolar II and Related Conditions," *Psychiatr Clin North Am*, 2002; 25(4): 713–37.

[11] DA Regier, WE Narrow, DS Rae, et al., "The De Facto Mental and Addictive Disorders Service System. Epidemiologic Catchment Area Prospective 1-Year Prevalence Rates of Disorders and Services," *Archives of General Psychiatry*, 1993; 50(2): 85–94.

Chapter 4

[1] E Frank, HA Swartz, and DJ Kupfer, "Interpersonal and Social Rhythm Therapy: Managing the Chaos of Bipolar Disorder," *Biol Psychiatry*, 2000 September 15; 48(6): 593–604. Review.

[2] S Malkoff-Schwartz, E Frank, B Anderson, et al., "Stressful Life Events and Social Rhythm Disruption in the Onset of Manic and Depressive Bipolar Episodes: A Preliminary Investigation," *Arch Gen Psychiatry*, 1998 August; 55(8): 702–7.

[3] R Sabatowski, D Schafer, S Kasper, et al., "Pain Treatment: A Historical Overview," *Current Pharmaceutical Design 10*, no. 7 (March 2004): 701–16.

[4] D Ford and D Kamerow, "Epidemiologic Study of Sleep Disturbances and Psychiatric Disorders. An Opportunity for Prevention?" *JAMA*, 1989 September 15; 262(11): 1479–84.

[5] T Overbeek, R van Diest, K Schruers, F Kruizinga, and E Griez, "Sleep Complaints in Panic Disorder Patients," *J Nerv Ment Dis*, 2005 July; 193(7): 488–93.

[6] HA Mansour, J Wood, KV Chowdari, et al., "Circadian Phase Variation in Bipolar I Disorder," *Chronobiol Int*, 2005; 22(3): 571–84.

[7] YH Wu and DF Swaab, "The Human Pineal Gland and Melatonin in Aging and Alzheimer's Disease," *J Pineal Res*, 2005 April; 38(3): 145–52.

[8] SH Jones, DJ Hare, and K Evershed, "Actigraphic Assessment of Circadian Activity and Sleep Patterns in Bipolar Disorder," *Bipolar Disord*, 2005 April; 7(2): 176.

[9] JT Arnedt, J Owens, and M Crouch, "Neurobehavioral Performance of Residents After Heavy Night Call vs After Alcohol Ingestion," *JAMA*, 2005; 294:1025–33.

[10] A Harvey, D Schmidt, A Scarna, et al., "Sleep-Related Functioning in Euthymic Patients with Bipolar Disorder, Patients with Insomnia, and Subjects without Sleep Problems," *Am J Psychiatry*, 2005; 162:50–57.

[11] RH Howland, "Sleep-Onset Rapid Eye Movement Periods in Neuropsychiatric Disorders: Implications for the Pathophysiology of Psychosis," *J Nerv Ment Dis*, 1997 December; 185(12): 730–38.

[12] GW Vogel, A Buffenstein, K Minter, and A Hennessey, "Drug Effects on REM Sleep and on Endogenous Depression," *Neurosci Biobehav Rev*, 1990; 14:49–63.

[13] JM Allen, RW Lam, RA Remick, and AD Sadovnick, "Depressive Symptoms and Family History in Seasonal and Nonseasonal Mood Disorders," *Am J Psychiatry*, 1993; 150:443–48.

[14] L Sher, "Alcoholism and Seasonal Affective Disorder," *Compr Psychiatry*, 2004 January–February; 45(1): 51–56. Review.

[15] AL Miller, "Epidemiology, Etiology, and Natural Treatment of Seasonal Affective Disorder," *Altern Med Rev*, 2005 March; 10(1): 5–13.

[16] Adapted from *American Psychiatric Association, Diagnostic and Statistical Manual of Mental Disorders*, 4th ed. (Washington, DC: American Psychiatric Association, 2000), 390.

[17] V Coiro, R Volpi, C Marchesi, and A De Ferri, "Abnormal Serotonergic Control of Prolactin and Cortisol Secretion in Patients with Seasonal Affective Disorder," *Psychoneuroendocrinology*, 1993; 18(8): 551–56.

[18] R Hakkarainen, C Johansson, and T Kieseppa, "Seasonal Changes, Sleep Length and Circadian Preference among Twins with Bipolar Disorder," *BMC Psychiatry*, 2003 June 9; 3(1): 6.

[19] B Sep-Kowalikowa, "Phototherapy as a Supporting Treatment in Depressive Patients," *Psychiatr Pol*, 2002 November–December; 36(6 Suppl): 99–108.

[20] NE Rosenthal, "Light Therapy: Theory and Practice," *Primary Psychiatry*, (September/October 1994):31.

[21] AM Ghadirian, BE Murphy, and MJ Gendron, "Efficacy of Light versus Tryptophan Therapy in Seasonal Affective Disorder," *J Affect Disord*, 1998 July; 50(1): 23–27.

[22] A Neumeister, N Praschak-Rieder, and B Hesselman, "Effects of Tryptophan Depletion in Fully Remitted Patients with Seasonal Affective Disorder during Summer," *Psychol Med*, 1998 March; 28(2): 257–64.

Chapter 5

[1] Surgeon General's Report on Mental Health, 1999.

[2] http://www.projo.com/extra/election/content/projo_20050331_joan31. 2525401. html.

[3] Jean-Claude Van Damme, interview, *Entertainment Weekly*, September 4, 1998.

[4] "Carrie Fisher: Perhaps One of Manic-Depression's Best-Known Champions, the Writer and Actress Shows Us How She Wrangles Her Many Moods." Interview by M Lybi. *Psychology Today*, November 1, 2001.

[5] "Celeb Life: 'My husband lived in fear of me' On screen, she was The Terminator's tough-as-nails Sarah Connor, but in real life, star Linda Hamilton was going through hell as she battled manic depression . . ." (Features) Sunday Mirror (London, England); January 16, 2005.

[6] RE Morehouse, F Farley, and JV Youngquist, "Type T Personality and the Jungian Classification System." *J Pers Assess*, 1990 Spring; 54(1–2): 231–35.

Chapter 6

[1] "Bipolar II Disorder and its Beneficial Subtype: A Desirable Disorder," by Ronald R. Fieve, MD, in Current Psychiatric Therapy, ed. David Dunner, MD, W.B. Saunders Company, 1997.

[2] John D. Gartner, *The Hypomanic Edge*, Simon & Schuster 2005.

[3] Ronald R. Fieve, MD. *Moodswing: Dr. Fieve on Depression*, William Morrow, 1975, 2nd Edition, Bantam Dell, 1997.

[4] Kay Redfield Jamison, *Exuberance*, Knopf, 2004.

[5] "Patient Rejection of Lithium Carbonate Prophylaxis," Philip Polatin, MD, & Ronald R. Fieve, MD, *Journal of the American Medical Association*, page 218, 1971, Nov. 18.

Chapter 7

[1] T Suppes, EB Dennehy, and EW Gibbons, "The Longitudinal Course of Bipolar Disorder," *J Clin Psychiatry*, 2000; 61 Suppl 9:23–30.

[2] BM McGrath, PH Wessels, EC Bell, M Ulrich, and PH Silverstone, "Neurobiological Findings in Bipolar II Disorder Compared with Findings in Bipolar I Disorder," *Can J Psychiatry*, 2004 December; 49(12): 794–801. Review.

Chapter 8

[1] R Larson, "Lithium Prevents Suicides," *Insights on the News*, 1998; 14 (18): 39.

[2] JR Calabrese, CL Bowden, GS Sachs, et al., "A Double-Blind Placebo-Controlled Study of Lomotrigine Monotherapy in Outpatients with Bipolar I Depression. Lamictal 602 Study Group," *Clin Psychiatry*, 1999; 60(2): 79, 88.

[3] JR Calabrese, T Suppes, CL Bowden, et al., "A Double-Blind, Placebo-Controlled Prophylaxis Study of Lamotrigine in Rapid-Cycling Bipolar Disorder. Lamictal 614 Study Group," *J Clin Psychiatry*, 2000; 61(11): 841–50.

[4] PE Keck, RH Perlis, MW Otto, et al. The Expert Consensus Guideline Series. *Treatment of Bipolar Disorder*, 2004. A Postgraduate Medicine Special Report. 2004(December): 41.

Chapter 9

[1] RC Kessler, PA Berglund, O Demler, R Jin, and EE Walters, "Lifetime Prevalence and Age-of-Onset Distributions of *DSM-IV* Disorders in the National Comorbidity Survey Replication (NCS-R)," *Archives of General Psychiatry*, 2005 June; 62(6): 593–602.

[2] M Steiner, "Postpartum Psychiatric Disorders," *Can J Psychiatry* 1990; 35:89.

[3] "Diagnostic Criteria for ADHD," in *Diagnostic and Statistical Manual of Mental Disorders*, 4th ed. (DSM-IV). (Washington, DC: American Psychiatric Association, 1994).

[4] National Institute of Mental Health, "Depression in Children and Adolescents," http://www.nimh.nih.gov/HealthInformation/depchildmenu.cfm.

[5] Modified from the National Institute of Mental Health's "Let's Talk Depression," NIH Publication, 01-4162, June 2001.

[6] American Academy of Child and Adolescent Psychiatry, "Facts for Families #10: Teen Suicide," http://www.aacap.org/publications/factsfam/suicide.htm.

[7] National Center for Chronic Disease Prevention and Health Promotion, Adolescent and School Health, Youth Risk Behavior Surveillance System (2001).

[8] RW Maris, "Suicide," *Lancet*, 2002 July 27; 360(9329): 319–26. Review.

Chapter 10

[1] D Miklowitz, "Psychosocial Factors in the Course and Treatment of Bipolar Disorder. The Future of Bipolar Disorder Mood Stabilization," *CME*, October 1, 2004.

[2] K Wilkins, "Bipolar I Disorder, Social Support and Work," *Health Rep*, 2004; 15 Suppl:21–30.

[3] JS House, KR Landis, and D Umberson, "Social Relationships and Health," *Science*, 1988; 241:541–45.

[4] S Maddi, "On Hardiness and Other Pathways to Resilience," *American Psychologist*, 2005; 60(3): 261–62.

[5] DJ Miklowitz, TL Simoneau, EL George, et al., "Family-Focused Treatment of Bipolar Disorder: 1-Year Effects of a Psychoeducational Program in Conjunction with Pharmacotherapy," *Biol Psychiatry*, 2000 September 15; 48(6): 582–92.

[6] PE Keck Jr., "Defining and Improving Response to Treatment in Patients with Bipolar Disorder," *J Clin Psychiatry*, 2004; 65 Suppl 15:25–29. Review.

[7] G Harvey, A Schmidt, A Scarna, et al., "Sleep-Related Functioning in Euthymic Patients with Bipolar Disorder, Patients with Insomnia, and Subjects without Sleep Problems," *Am J Psychiatry*, 2005 January; 162:50–57.

INDEX

Underscored page references indicate boxed text. **Boldface** references indicate illustrations.

in children and adolescents,
220–21, 222
compulsive spending with,
124–25
decreased sleep needs with,
22–23, 46, 48, 71–72,
86, 87, 88, 97
downside of, 23–26
DSM-IV criteria for, 48–50
energy misidentified as, 181
gambling with, 125–26
hypersexuality with, 111–13,
115–16, 117, **118**
vs. mania, 18, 21
resistance to treatment of,
26
from seasonal affective
disorder, 102–3
substance abuse with, 120,
128
symptoms of, 5, 6, 17–21, 24,
46–50, 47, 55, 58, 112,
235
in teens, 220–21
treatment of, 16–17, 26, 113,
182
unipolar, 40
upside of, 21–23, 29
use of term, 7
Hypomanic advantage of bipolar
IIB, 10, 11, 29, 130–32
Hypomanic alert, 9
Hypothymic temperament,
63–64, 235
Hypothyroidism, 27, 176–77,
177–78

I

Immediate gratification, from
risky behaviors, 127
Impulsivity
with ADHD, 217
risky behaviors from, 128

Insomnia
with bipolar disorder, 95,
98–99
with major depression, 88
prevalence of, 89
as sign of psychiatric disorder,
92
symptoms of, 98
Interpersonal and Social Rhythm
Therapy, 241–42
Interpersonal Psychotherapy, 241
Intuitive and captivating
behavior, in bipolar IIB,
150–51
Irregular sleep-wake schedule, 100

K

Kennedy family, 121, 144
Kidder, Margot, 151
Kleptomania, 128
Klonopin (clonazepam), 191

L

Laboratory tests
for diagnosis and treatment,
177–78
for ruling out physical
conditions, 162–63
Lamictal (lamotrigine), 189–90,
190–91, 200
for adolescents, 224
expert consensus on, 197
Letourneau, Mary Kay, 109–10
Lexapro (escitalopram oxalate),
37
Light therapy
for delayed sleep phase
syndrome, 99
for seasonal affective disorder,
105–6
Limbaugh, Rush, 141
Lincoln, Abraham, 144–45

Selective serotonin reuptake
inhibitors (SSRIs), 36–37,
38, <u>195</u>
suicide and, 224–25
Self-advocacy, for accurate
diagnosis, 170–74
Self-help strategies
for bipolar families, <u>85</u>
for bipolar II disorder, <u>30</u>
for bipolar IIB, <u>153</u>
for medication use, <u>205</u>
for obtaining diagnosis, <u>180</u>
for risky behaviors, <u>129</u>
for sleep problems, <u>108</u>
in specific situations, 230–31
for staying well, <u>249</u>
for understanding bipolar
spectrum, <u>64</u>
Self-Rating Mood Scale, 233,
<u>234–35</u>
Seroquel (quetiapine), 189, 191,
197, <u>201</u>
Serotonin
carbohydrates increasing, 101
drugs increasing, 35, 36
mood disorders and, 34–35,
36, 38, 105
in neurobiology of suicide, <u>223</u>
Serotonin Only Hypothesis,
37–38
Serotonin-norepinephrine
reuptake inhibitors
(SNRIs), 38, <u>195</u>
Serzone (nefazodone), 37
Sexual compulsivity or addiction.
See also Hypersexuality
characteristics of, 113–16
harmful effects of, 116–17
hypomania leading to, **118**
questions for recognizing,
117–18
Sleep
antipathy toward, in bipolar
IIB, 146–47

average need for, 89
circadian rhythms and, 90,
93–95, 99
history of research on,
90–92
normal, 92
stages of, 91–92, 95–96
Sleep deprivation, effects of,
97–98
Sleep medications, <u>193</u>
Sleep needs
decreased
with bipolar disorder,
89–90
with hypomania, 22–23,
46, 48, 71–72, 86, 87,
88, 97
with mania, 43, 88
increased, with bipolar II
depression, 88
Sleep problems
delayed sleep phase syndrome,
99
with depression, 95, 96–97,
98, 99–100
hypersomnia, 92, 95
insomnia, 88, 89, 92, 95,
98–99
irregular sleep-wake schedule,
100
misdiagnosis of, 96
as presented in *Bipolar II*, 9
REM sleep abnormalities,
99–100
resolving, as stay-well strategy,
246–47, <u>249</u>
self-help for, <u>108</u>
signs of, <u>91</u>
studies on, 89–90
SNRI. *See* Serotonin-
norepinephrine reuptake
inhibitors
Social rhythm disruptions, 89–90,
242

RONALD R. FIEVE, MD

Internationally renowned psychiatrist and psychopharmacologist Ronald R. Fieve, MD, is *the* pioneer in the use of lithium for bipolar illness in America. A graduate of Harvard Medical School, extensively trained in psychopharmacology and psychiatry, he served his residencies at New York Hospital in internal medicine, and in psychiatry at the New York State Psychiatric Institute at Columbia Presbyterian Medical Center, Columbia University, New York City. Dr. Fieve is professor of clinical psychiatry at Columbia Presbyterian Medical Center; chief of research, department of lithium studies at the New York State Psychiatric Institute; and currently president and executive director of the Foundation for Mood Disorders in New York City.

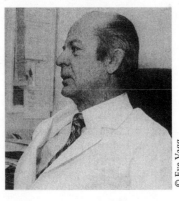

© Eve Vagg

He is the author of the best-selling book, *Moodswing: Dr. Fieve on Depression,* as well as *Prozac: Questions and Answers for Patients, Families, and Physicians* and *Second Opinion on Lithium Therapy for Depression and Manic-Depression.*

Dr. Fieve serves on the editorial boards of two French scientific journals, *L'Encephale* and *Lithium,* and has published more than 300 articles in scientific journals. He's also had many television appearances and countless speaking engagements in the United States and abroad.

Dr. Fieve maintains his private practice and Fieve Clinical Services (FCS) research office at 952 Fifth Avenue in Manhattan, directed and managed by his two daughters, an attorney and a psychologist. In this setting, Dr. Fieve and his associates evaluate and treat private patients, carry out second opinion consultations, serve as expert witnesses in legal cases, and conduct "no fee" clinical trials on new drugs under development in the pharmaceutical industry.